Drawn from Memory

A Personal Story of Healing through Art

E.J. Cockey

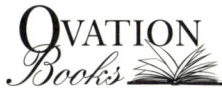

DRAWN FROM MEMORY: A PERSONAL STORY OF HEALING THROUGH ART
PUBLISHED BY OVATION BOOKS
P.O. Box 80107
AUSTIN, TX 78758

For more information about our books, please write to us, call 512.478.2028, or visit our website at www.ovationbooks.net.

Printed and bound in China. All rights reserved. No part of this book may be reproduced in any form or by any electronic or mechanical means including information storage and retrieval systems without permission in writing from the copyright holder, except by a reviewer, who may quote brief passages in review.

Distributed to the trade by National Book Network, Inc.

Library of Congress Cataloging-in-Publication available upon request.

ISBN-13: 978-0-9790275-1-2
ISBN-10: 0-9790275-1-9

Copyright© 2007 E.J. Cockey

A portion of the proceeds will be donated to Good Samaritan Nursing Center in Baltimore, Maryland. For more information about Good Samaritan Hospital's programs and services, including its long-term care program and nursing center, visit their website at http://www.goodsam-md.org.

Prologue

This is a true story about my life and the lives of those I know. Some are still with me, and some have passed away — although not everyone who passed has necessarily died. I think it's always hardest in the beginning to intuit how things are going to go; as for myself, I have been fooled many times.

Nonetheless I have seen fit to change the names of everyone appearing in this story, and in some cases I've made slight identity changes to protect innocent people. I have also changed or omitted names of institutions, hospitals, and long-term care facilities.

I remember when my mother had to go into a nursing facility; every time I visited she cried and clung to me, begging me to stay longer. Then she'd ask me to take her home. "Please don't leave me by myself," she repeated. Over the years, I have heard this from many long-term patients, even though their histories and afflictions are quite different. They just want to go home again. I have listened and comforted many dying people and have distilled what they told me into three basic questions. I feel that these questions are central to our lives and that it is unfortunate when a person hasn't addressed them long before he or she faces a debilitating illness or death:

1. Am I going to suffer?
2. Will I be alone?
3. Did my life mean something?

Pondering these questions and being willing to answer them has made a vast difference to me over the last several years. People who were dying have taught me more about living than any other source ever did, and for this I will always be grateful. I also learned that good does not come to those who deserve it, but to those who are ready for it, and I discovered that suffering is not an inevitable part of life.

But let me explain before I go any further. My story will make more sense if I supply some sort of context to hang it on. Writing is a lot like the art I do with dementia patients. I give them a context by drawing a line to form a particular shape: It could be a house, a tree, a vase, or the street below. That way it's always clear what I'm talking about. A tree is a tree, after all!

About 13 years ago, I started working as an art teacher for several long-term care facilities. Since that time I have earned my master's degree in art therapy. At first I worked with dementia patients only; later I expanded my art programs to include others with special needs.

I'm one of the people who care for the individuals our society has cast aside: the ones who need us the most — the dying, the infirm, and the meek.

The story I'm telling lies in the experience we had together. Me on the outside, looking in. Them on the inside, pushing out. In retrospect, I think I have brought laughter to them, but what they have given me is much greater. I found out that we are not equal, none of us. Some ride in wheelchairs, others can't see. Many are crippled and incontinent, with leaky brains, dead limbs, and useless bodies. They are multicolored. Some are still young, most are very old. Many are forgotten. The truth is we are all uniquely different; none of us is the same. But what they have taught me is that we are something far more important than *equal*.

We are all in this together.

Amazing grace! (how sweet the sound)
That sav'd a wretch like me!
I once was lost, but now am found,
Was blind, but now I see…
Thro' many dangers, toils and snares,
I have already come,
'Tis grace has brought me safe thus far,
And grace will lead me home.

Rev. John Newton

1779 Edition of Olney Hymns
Harry Ransom Humanities Research Center
University of Texas at Austin

Chapter 1

April 16, 2004

It was a beautiful day. Cumulous clouds floated high in a bright blue sky as we drove along the old dirt road. My real estate agent, Connie, was driving, and I was sitting on the passenger side. I had rolled down the window so that I could guide her past some thistles growing right up to the roadway's edge. On the left we could see the Ondawa River, full with brown swirling water from last night's storm. Connie is my best friend from childhood. We grew up in the same town and have known each other since kindergarten. The reason for our drive that spring day? I had decided to sell the 16 acres of pristine riverfront I'd inherited from my parents. I had owned the property for several years but visited only once in all that time.

Connie stopped the car at the end of the dirt road. Before us, a stretch of pasture grew all the way along one side of the river for a quarter-mile or so. She looked at me, then past me toward the river. I already knew what she was going to say.

"Why are you selling this?" she asked.

"I'm tired of paying the taxes," I answered. I looked at the river, too. Along the bank on either side grew tall pines. I had played there as a child, fished along those same banks for trout, dug under the rocks for crayfish. The trees were stately, and they

cast deep shadows across the stream. "It's so pretty," Connie said. "You could paint a picture of it."
"I've got plenty of pictures of it, " I said. "I hate it, actually. This property isn't really mine. I inherited it by default."
"What do you mean?" she asked.
I twisted in the front seat to face her. The river was to my back. I could feel a cold breeze through the open window. I shivered in spite of the fact that the sun was shining and the day was warm. "My parents built their dream house down here on this property because they loved that river," I said. "But they never realized the dream. It was over almost before they had moved into the house."
"You can always start over again," Connie said. "It's all still here."
"And therein lies the problem," I said. "I would love to call this place home, but it's not. It's only filled with bad memories that I would just as soon forget."
Connie sighed. She began pulling papers out of her briefcase. "Let's get on with it then," she said. "I've got other comparative listings here. I think you can get a pretty good price."
"How much do you think it's worth?" I asked.
"About eighty-five thousand, give or take," she replied.
I was drifting. My mind had wandered off to another time, another day on the banks of this river. Suddenly I was remembering the barbecue. My parents had invited what seemed like the entire town. The barbecue was also their housewarming party; relatives had driven or flown in for the weekend. I had driven up from Baltimore with the boys for the festivities.

June 24, 1990

It was dusk. The party had been going on for hours. It had been a full day. I'd visited with old high school buddies and townsfolk; now I was tired. I stood in a pasture that led down to the river. My father had mowed it the day before. He had also built a huge fire pit fashioned from ancient, crumbling stone walls. The fire pit had been the main attraction, but after it started to smoke, the crowd had moved away from it. Now the Ondawa River had captured my attention since I had walked down toward the water with the rest. It was serene and lovely, there in the fading light. The last rays of the sun filtered down onto the water, forming patterns. Tiny lightning bugs had come out, too numerous to count, their little lights repeating, reflecting a thousand times on the river as it flowed by.

There were more than a hundred people gathered along the river's edge — townsfolk, friends, and family. I'd been answering questions about my recent divorce and future plans. I had grown tired of these personal questions, especially since they involved talking about my failed marriage. I was exhausted and trying to visually locate my two boys. I didn't know where they were. I scanned the river again. They had wandered off to catch crayfish some time ago. Fourteen-year-old Ben was supposed to be in charge of his younger brother Gray, who was seven. I really didn't trust the older one to take care of his brother, but he was my only choice at the time. This had added to my sense of remorse about my ex-husband.

I could hear my father calling, "Last chance to get your meat on the grill!"

Already people were shifting about, starting to gather their things. It would soon be time to cut the cake and sing one more song before the party was officially over. I could see my boys now, clambering up the bank. Ben carried a pail, presumably holding crayfish, and Gray followed close behind. Even from a distance I could see that they were covered with mud up to their knees, and I groaned silently.

"What's the matter with you?"

I turned to see my brother walking toward me. He was carrying a card table in one hand and two chairs in the other. I was amazed at his strength and dexterity. He stopped directly in front of me, putting the chairs down first. "What's up with you?" he asked.

"Are you talking to me?" I asked.

"Yes, you looked really weird just now standing there all by yourself," he said. "Is something wrong?" As he talked, he set the table down by the chairs, dusted off his hands, and stood waiting for me to respond.

"Just tired, that's all," I replied. "It's been a long day."

"Well it's almost over, he said. "Once we find out where Mom's gotten off to, we're ready to start cutting the cake." He turned toward the river and put his hand up to shield his eyes from the sun's fading light.

"I don't see her." he said. "Do you know where she might have gone?"

I shrugged. "The last time I talked with her it was about an hour ago, and she looked all done in. I told her to sit down, but she didn't, of course," I said.

My brother frowned. "I thought she looked more tired than usual too," he said.

"Well, they've had a long week, moving furniture into the new house and then preparing for this party. Mom probably did most of the cooking. And she's *old*," I added for emphasis. He shook his head in agreement.

"You're probably right." he said. "I'm going to look in the house though, because Dad wants to wrap this party up soon. Why don't you ask your kids? Maybe they've seen her."

"All right," I said, and went to find the boys. They'd been heading toward the picnic tables with their catch.

"Gray, Ben," I cried. "Come here. I want to ask you something."

Gray dropped his pail in the newly mowed grass and started running. Ben, being older and faster, quickly overtook him, and they came to a screeching halt right in front of me, nearly knocking me off my feet. I stepped back from them, laughing and catching my breath.

"We caught lots of crawdads in the river, Momma," Gray said.

"It's crawfish, stupid," Ben said.

At this remark, Gray made a fist, which I intercepted rather deftly. Holding his hand in the air and away from Ben, I asked them if they had seen Grandma.

"She was wading in the river when we came back," Ben replied. "I think she said she was going to wade all the way across to the other side."

"Gramma said she was looking for something," Gray said.

"What was she looking for?" I asked.

I never did find out exactly why my mother waded into the river that day or what she had said to Gray. Our conversation was ended abruptly by a loud scream. The three of us turned and looked in the direction of the sound. It had come from the river. Suddenly everyone was running at once, overturning chairs, and spilling drinks in the way. The boys and I made it down to the bank. I could hear the water lapping up along the edge as I stood there with the others. In the distance I could see my high school friend, Sam Perkins, pulling someone out of the river. He was yelling to his wife, Emily.

"Call the emergency squad," he was screaming.

My father was there, too. He had reached the water's edge about the same time as Sam. Now I could hear him yelling and sobbing. "Oh my God," he cried.

I pushed my way past several people to see who had been dragged to the shore. My heart sank as I came closer to my father and Sam. My mother lay motionless between them. Sam was pulling her over onto her back, holding her nose, and breathing into her mouth. He repeated this maneuver several times. Suddenly she became rigid, then her body arched backward, and foam came from her mouth.

"What's happening to her?" my father cried. He looked panic-stricken in the fading light.

Meanwhile, Sam turned again to ask if anyone had called the emergency squad. As a crowd, we had become immobilized; no one seemed to be able to go anywhere.

Finally in the distance I heard a siren, then I could see the ambulance racing along the driveway, past the house, and finally into the field that had been our party ground. I don't remember how we all got home or what the boys did with their crayfish. It's all a blur. In the end, all I can remember is the sound of my father crying.

July 10, 1990

Later that same summer I stood with my mother in the cereal aisle at the Grand Union grocery in my home town. She was looking for a particular kind of granola, and we were faced with what seemed like hundreds of choices. The problem was that she couldn't tell me what she wanted — she was unable to speak.

I pointed to various boxes of granola. "What do you think about the kind with raisins?" I asked. Of course she didn't say anything, so I tried again to get her attention.

"*Mom*, are you listening?"

Again, no response, and then I remembered that she couldn't speak since her accident in the river. I wasn't used to this scenario yet, but I was hoping she could still communicate with me. I was fairly certain that she could at least hear what I was saying. I turned to look at her directly, but when I looked around and saw that she wasn't there, I had to suppress my panic.

I looked down the aisle to see if Mom was anywhere in sight, and I spied her. She was standing by the dairy case, picking up yogurt and cottage cheese. Mom had taken several containers of each and was carefully placing them into someone else's cart. Our own cart was still behind me.

"Good Lord!" I said. She looked up from the stranger's cart, saw me, pointed in my direction, and started giggling. I turned around to see what she was pointing at. It was her closest neighbor, Jean Brown, approaching us. My mother's affliction was not something my family wanted everybody in town to find out about just yet. We were hoping that eventually things would just get back to normal. This was a secret that we had decided to keep, and right now it was up to me to maintain security.

It would be worse still for Mrs. Brown to find out about

my mother's problem. In my opinion, she had really missed her calling by not writing a gossip column for the local newspaper.

So I put on my happiest face and smiled at her as she maneuvered her cart my way. Mrs. Brown ignored me completely and walked down the isle toward my mother. "How are you Annette?" she said. "I heard you were in the hospital!"

Mom was still giggly, but she didn't respond to Mrs. Brown, which was a great relief. Instead of saying anything, she pushed the cart she had been putting yogurt into around the corner and disappeared behind a display of canned goods. I couldn't believe it! How was I ever going to keep this situation a secret? And how did Mrs. Brown find out about my mother so soon? Before I could think about a reasonable excuse for my mom's behavior, Mrs. Brown had moved closer to me. In a hushed voice, she asked me for details. Her eyes were wide with surprise and delight.

"What was the prognosis?" she whispered.

"Gee, I don't know. The jury's still out," I lied. My brain was working fast now to come up with a reasonable excuse she would believe. "But poor Mom caught something while she was in the hospital, and now she's got laryngitis. I think she's a bit confused with all the commotion," I said. "She's not supposed to be using her voice today." I added this as an afterthought.

"That's terrible!"

Mrs. Brown's face was all scrunched, as if she were thinking hard, and I could tell that she was sizing my story up, wondering what to do with this information. I waited, thinking that she would begin to interrogate me if I hung around any longer. But she didn't say anything, and I felt more confident that I had managed to stay on top of the situation.

"Well, stay in touch," she said, "and don't be a stranger."

"I'm only here for a few more days," I said.

To indicate that our conversation had reached a conclusion, I pushed my cart around Mrs. Brown, making a beeline for the canned goods. Luckily I found my mother there, examining cans of peas.

"Let's get out of here," I pleaded. "Please Mom, before anyone else sees us!" I think I must have surprised her. What she did next haunts me to this very day. Mother began to cry, loudly enough that everyone around us could hear her. Tears ran down her face.

"Let's go home," I said frantically. "Let's just forget the damned cereal." She stopped crying for a moment as if she were pondering this, and then reached out to clutch my hand. She has never liked it when I get upset. Fortunately we were able to make our way out the door like that, abandoning the cart, with me holding onto her arm and her hand clutching mine. I managed to propel her like that toward the lot where I had parked the car. It was difficult and awkward. It was hot, and the sun was bearing down.

I thought that I should say something that might calm her and that indirectly would calm me too, which is how I came to say to her that it was going to be all right somehow. "It's going to be OK, this is nothing! Why I've seen worse than this!" I said.

When my parents had retired earlier that year, they had decided to build their dream house down by the river on some property that had been part of the family farm. The land hadn't been farmed for at least a generation, so the riverfront property was an ideal location for a peaceful way of life. Their new home was a rustic cabin, with a cedar deck around it. From every direction came a chorus of animal sounds. They were going to be happy there, they had planned it that way. But it didn't work out the way they planned.

Mother was always an active person and hoped to stay that way by exercising on a daily basis. Her favorite activity was swimming, and she loved the idea of living next to the river. Apparently she had waded into the river, suffered a grand mal seizure, and gone under. A CAT scan revealed angiomas in her brain, little knots of abnormal blood vessels that had caused the seizure and consequently her loss of speech and the slight dementia.

Despite all this, the doctor was reassuring. "Don't worry. In a few days she'll be right as rain," he said.

He had sent my mother home with a bottle of anti-seizure medication and told her to relax. It took another year and many more tests and trips to the hospital before we found out the final diagnosis. Mother had been born with a rare hereditary disease: familial cerebral angiomatosis disease. The lesions in her brain had grown larger as she had grown older. On the day of the party, one of those lesions ruptured in the left frontal lobe, robbing her of speech. Eventually these same lesions also robbed her of a relationship with my father, their dream house on the river, and the ability to take care of herself.

To his credit, my father took care of her all by himself in their new house for the next five years. When questioned about this decision, he replied, "I promised I wouldn't send her to a nursing home." One day she fell in the bathroom while he was out shopping, and lay helpless for several hours until my father came home to find her. She had gotten herself wedged between the toilet and the wall. Their dog, Yankee, was licking her face. Wet, confused, and frightened, she didn't even recognize my father.

She doesn't remember me at all now, or any of us for that matter: my sister and brother, our children, or her friends. She was moved to the Alzheimer's unit last spring. The doctor has told me not to telephone her any more because it upsets her and she cries. She thinks I am coming to take her home again.

But home is just not the same without her being there, so I don't visit more than twice a year. I don't like to admit it, but I just can't stand it. When I do visit, I have to see her in the special care unit at Community Convalescent Nursing Facility. It is devastating to see her in a wheelchair, not to be able to talk with her, and finally, to leave her behind when I go. The last time I saw my mother, all she said was this: "Don't leave me here!"

Chapter 2

The hospital has a nursing facility behind the main building, making it a campus of sorts. It is one of my favorite places to practice art therapy. The activity room where all this art takes place is on the second floor. Tall windows on three sides of the building look out onto a tree-lined street below. There is ample light and lots of space to move wheelchairs around without bumping into anything. Appropriately, it's called the Park Unit. If you are deaf, Park Unit is a good place to hang out during the day. Otherwise, with the noise level and the constant sounds, both mechanical and human, you could really consider being deaf an asset. There are bells ringing and beepers beeping and little old ladies and men strapped into wheelchairs and narrow beds. They stare up at the ceiling and repeat the same things over and over and over all day long, every day, perpetually.

"Mommy, mommy, mommy, mommy ..." one woman cries.

March 18, 2004

I step off the elevator and turn right at the doors. Alex has already set up the room by moving tables together and covering them with plastic cloths. Several nursing aides help Alex move the patients around the room and into place at the tables as I arrive. For at least another five minutes there is a bustle of activity, and once everyone is rounded up, there are 16 people ready to begin art class. I work more or less with the same group every week. Sometimes a person dies, but that's about the only reason they don't show up on a regular basis to paint with me.

They are bored.

Truth be told, there's not a lot of activities you can do with a mixed group of people suffering from a wide variety of diseases such as Parkinson's, Alzheimer's, dementia, and multiple sclerosis. There are also other special-needs residents here: amputees, diabetics, and quadriplegics. I never know exactly who I'll have each week or what kind of emotional condition they'll be in, either.

The reason I came to Park Unit in the first place was to see if I could help this group of residents because they were clinically depressed. The reason they were depressed was because they were spending the rest of their lives on Park Unit, minus arms and legs and minds. However, the real problem wasn't related to the illnesses as much as it was to the fact that they were all having rather normal reactions to their monotonous and institutionalized living conditions.

"Let's do art!" I announce as I walk to the end of one of the tables and wait for their attention.

I stand next to Betty, who lost a leg last year to diabetes and has been in a wheelchair ever since. She is wearing a bright green plastic party hat left over from a St. Patrick's Day celebration the night before. One hand is strapped down to her wheelchair in some kind of foam contraption. In the other hand she holds a short stick with a coat hook attached by duct tape to one end. Betty eyeballs me from her ground position and gets a look on her face that tells me something's coming.

"Git her outta here!" she bellows, and points to Mary, who is sitting a couple of seats down from her.

"Hey," I say "what's up with the big stick, Betty? Aren't they feeding you this week?" This comment brings laughter from Betty's end of the table. Then I turn to the person Betty is enraged with, a lady of undeterminable age, also in a wheelchair. I tend to agree with Betty that this lady is, in her terms, a total pain to deal with. She always has a headache.

"Hey, Mary, how are you today?"

"I can't find my glasses, and my head hurts so much that I can't paint," Mary whines.

"Knock it off, Mary," I say. "You never can find your glasses. Why heck, I don't think you even own glasses!" Several of the other patients laugh at this, too, and a lady named Helen tells me that Mary is definitely lying.

"I do have glasses, but *she* probably took them." Mary sneers and points at Betty.

"She was *born* with a headache!"

"Was not!"

And so it goes.

Sitting next to Mary is a gentleman named Darren. He is 79 years old and suffers from advanced dementia. I first met Darren four years ago. He was sitting in the same seat that he occupies now, only now he is looking around the room and smiling, waiting patiently to become the next person I "pick on." He likes to reminisce about the time he started painting with me. We go over this scenario every week or so.

I put my hand on his shoulder. "Hey buddy, what's up?"

"Stop messin with me," Darren says.

"I'm here *especially* to mess with you!" I remind him.

"Remember when I threw that brush?"

"Of course I do. You threw that brush three or four times across this room, and I picked it up every time and handed it back to you."

"And then I painted the pumpkin,"

"And you haven't stopped painting yet!"

Darren smiles and looks down at his hands. Actually, Darren sat at the activity table for a couple of years, refusing to do anything. He didn't interact with others, and he didn't like to be disturbed. He preferred to sit facing the tall windows. Trouble was that he didn't even look out at the scenery, but sat with his face tilted down all day and every day. Apparently the art class was the first social program that had any effect upon him at all.

Betty has just maneuvered her electric wheelchair into place at the head of the table. She is the alpha female at Park Unit; she is also my favorite. I just love her stick with the coat hanger on the end. She invented the contraption to push the button on the elevator since her hands don't reach it from the wheelchair. She's a survivor.

"Come here," she calls to me.

"What now?" I ask.

"I gotta tell you sompin what I said." She has that gleam in her eye, and I wonder what story she has for me this time. Usually her language and manner are rather crude, but she has a wonderful sense of humor. I look around the unit as I make my way over to her, checking to see if any family members are hanging around or anyone else who might get offended by what I anticipate will be a graphic description. She grabs hold of my arm and pulls me down until my head is on the same level as hers.

"Wanna know what I told the aide at lunch today?" she asks. She sits back and waits for me to respond. There is a naughty look on her face now.

"No, what?"

"So, I told her, you git over here and take this lousy sandwich back to the kitchen. You smelled this thing, I said to her? And she says she ain't smelt nothing today cause she's so busy. So I says to her, well you just git your nose down here, cause I'm telling you this thing smells worse than my toilet does!" She sits back in her chair laughing and waiting for my reaction.

I whisper into her ear, cupping my hand around that side of her head so no one else will hear. "You really need to find more to do around here."

"Trouble is, there ain't nothin round here worth doing." she says. Betty laughs again loudly and then raps her stick on the table. This is the signal that the class should come to order. She does this every week; it's a ritual. All 16 sets of eyes are on me.

"Let's paint, folks."

The next phase is all about movement and confusion mixed in with a little patience, some fighting, and a lot of laughter. Let me explain. There are always 15 to 20 individuals present for the art class, and they have clustered around the tables with some space in between, so that I can squeeze in between them. Generally they have a tendency not to socialize with one another unless they are playing bingo.

There are other people assisting me today: Alex, the activity aide; Chris, my personal assistant; Sister Maria, a Sister of Charity. Usually we're joined by a random family member, and today there are two men — William and Stan — flanking a lady named Ernestine. I can tell by their faces that they desperately want Ernestine to participate in this activity. She's new to the Park Unit, and it's very normal for people's families to want to get them off to a great start. It eases the pain they feel when they have to go home and leave Grandma or their spouse behind.

"Why don't you stay where you are and paint with her?"

"You sure it wouldn't be no trouble?" William asks. "I'm her husband."

"Of course it's not. I'll have Alex bring you some paper."

Alex is already handing out white paper to everyone, and Chris is distributing paint brushes. I head for the paint cart and begin to squirt different colors into small plastic drinking cups. Betty is working on an outdoor scene with azaleas in bloom, only Chris has given her the wrong color, and she has painted a stream in with gray instead of light blue.

"This looks like shit," she complains.

"Hold tight Betty, I'll be right with you," I reply.

I decide to give Sue the blue paint first. She is sitting on Betty's right and has a big sky area that could be filled in nicely with this particular hue. I decide that Betty can use it in a minute. They will have to learn how to share. Instead Sue looks up at me and whines, "I hate that color."

"Knock it off, Sue; this is an awesome color for that sky."

She begrudgingly takes the cup and starts to fill in the top of her painting, a landscape. "I want to paint a horse instead," she says.

"OK, but not now," I tell her.

Mary is next. Her arms are crossed, and she announces that she's only watching today. "I've got a bad headache today," she says.

"That's wonderful, darling!"

"My stomach hurts too!"

I know that she is only saying this because she needs the attention. I give her one of my stern looks while Alex hands her a cup of red paint. I am not trying to be unsympathetic to anyone. But this is therapy, and they are here to begin using arms and hands again. Talking and laughter come next, sometimes in a few weeks, usually in several months, but they always come.

For this I give thanks.

This activity lasts an hour and a half. I had to increase the time from the typical hour I usually allow for disabled individuals. There were so many people who wanted to paint that we scarcely had time to give everyone the attention they deserved. It would seem as if we had just gotten started before it would be quitting time. I talked the director of activities into adding some extra time, and now everybody gets what they need: attention! In fact, Alex has told me that my art class is as popular as bingo.

Finally they settle down, and everyone is painting, with the exception of Rosie, who is sleeping, slumped over in her wheelchair, but she's still holding onto a brush full of brown paint. I sigh. I'm tired, and everyone seems moody today. I look up to see what time it is; already 45 minutes have gone by.

Where does the time go?

I stare out the windows for a moment, hearing the traffic sounds on Smith Avenue: cars braking, horns blowing, and people calling to each other down below. The yelling reminds me of another time, and I begin to drift off in my mind while I gaze out the windows.

August 10, 1956

The main thing I remember about my grandmother: She was the ruling monarch of our family. My family's feeling of security depended upon her. She was a devout Baptist and generally opposed to the enjoyment of life's pleasures. Grandmother abstained from many things — the consumption of alcohol, playing cards, wearing makeup, touching, dancing, singing, laughing ... et cetera. She felt that it was her job to see to it that none of us strayed too far from the arms of Jesus! Poor Grandmother had been an adult since she was about nine years old. Her own mother, Sarah, was sickly and took to her bed about 1904. So the running of the house, cooking for the men, cleaning, and looking after her little brother, Collins, filled up Fanny's days, nights, and the remainder of her childhood years.

Sarah, on the other hand, became a painter, who had somehow managed to study art with a Hudson River School enthusiast. She painted in oils, hooked rag rugs, and allegedly received love poems from secret admirers. I inherited one of Sarah's oil paintings, which hangs over my dresser, and a love note written to her about 135 years ago. I guess it's pretty easy to see why Fanny, for her part, could have developed the belief that if anything was fun, you probably shouldn't be doing it. She didn't want to worry about going to hell, but the truth is, she really never had the time to go anyway.

One gray and moody August afternoon I had climbed up on top of the kitchen counter where I could sit in the large enameled sink. I was five years old. The sink was directly in front of the kitchen window, giving me a great view of the barn. I was looking at the barn, my face pressed to the glass, thinking about horses and horses in the barn! My grandfather had promised to buy me a horse when I was old enough, and I daydreamed about riding them all the time. I was leaning against the window where I could see the barn and dreaming about how my very own horse would live there someday. In a minute or two I would witness that barn being hit by lightning.

Suddenly the birds stopped chirping, and the wind came up, blowing dust from the driveway. The sky was starting to turn a hue of dark green, as if night were coming. The wind continued to pick up momentum and blew more dust across the driveway in front of our house, making it harder for me to see.

Then I heard a loud *boom* and saw a long streak of electricity leap out and reach right down into the top of the barn, followed by an immense *crack* and then another *boom*! Flames roared up and out of the roof. The lightning had struck the haymow, and the barn was burning! The next thing I saw was my grandfather running across the lawn. He was wearing his tall black rubber boots. I called them his shit-kicker boots because he always wore them to muck out the calf stalls. I remember wondering why he had those boots on. I just didn't see what difference they would make to a fire. He was screaming to my father, who followed close behind him. "Get moving, the barn is on fire!"

My father followed right behind him in the mad race toward the barn, and he was carrying a three-pronged hay fork. This gave him a similar appearance to a picture I had seen recently in Sunday school, a picture of Lucifer, the devil. Given the fact that my father was in possession of this pitchfork and was racing toward the fire gave me cause to feel uncertain and become frightened. I decided to remain at the window to see what was going to happen, mostly because the adults never told me anything. I was a kid.

Meanwhile, a different kind of calamity had taken over our household. My stalwart grandmother had come completely undone. She was running all over the place crying, carrying on, and upsetting everyone. My mother was hysterical, my baby brother was crying, and my little sister was whining that she was hungry. But I had remained at my perch on the kitchen sink where I had an extremely good view of the fire and the goings-on. I was yet unnoticed and hadn't been missed by the adults in all the excitement. Phone calls must have been made, though, because it wasn't too long before the townspeople began to arrive. They'd come either to help or to watch the 150-year-old barn burn to the ground. Pretty soon the driveway and then the front lawn had filled up with cars. Before too long, our house was surrounded by a parking lot! Some of the farm women had come along with their husbands and had found my grandmother sobbing on the steps, just under my window perch.

"We're ruined!" my grandmother cried.

I remember five or six women hovering around her, much like a football team would gather for a huddle with their quarterback. All heads were pointed toward the ground. I suppose that they were praying for the barn to stop burning. Eventually our minister, the Reverend Charles Plummer, appeared in the midst of this group of ladies. He was carrying two juice glasses half-full of a light-brown liquid. Reverend Plummer pulled up a lawn chair and sat directly in front of my grandmother, who was starting to cry again and rocking herself silly.

"Fanny Barber," he said, "you are going to pull yourself together now, and we are going to pray." She kept right on sobbing, though. He tried again.

"Here, sit up and drink this down," he commanded her. She looked up and took the juice glass from his hand.

"Just wha ... what am I d-drink-drinking?" she sobbed.

"It's medicine for the soul," he said.

She sniffed the contents of the glass and sat up straight. Her voice was suddenly commanding again "Oh, law, it's alcohol, the work of the devil!" she cried.

The next thing he told her has stuck with me since that very day. "Sometimes we just have to make exceptions," was what he said. Then the good Reverend Plummer drained his glass in one long gulp. He set the glass down on the lawn and waited.

"Am I going to go to hell for drinking this?"

Her hand was shaking, and some of the liquid was spilling out. He steadied her hand. "If you think you're going to hell, then I'm going right there with you, Fanny," he said. So she took a breath, and she drank the stuff all the way down.

"You are *crazy*!" was all she said afterward.

March 18, 2004

Suddenly I am brought back to the present because my cell phone is ringing. I normally don't take calls during a class, but when I look down I see it's the Professor calling. It seems odd that he would be calling me in the middle of the afternoon, so I answer the phone.

"This is Jack. I'm sorry to call you now, but I wanted you to know that Gertrude has had a stroke and is in the hospital," he said. I didn't respond immediately, because this news had caught me off-balance. I really didn't know what to say. Gertrude was my favorite old lady, and I felt like a part of her family. We had been together for more than five years.

"It doesn't seem to have affected her speech, but one side of her face has gone limp, and we're not sure if she can see out of one eye," he said.

I found my voice. "Where is she now?" I asked.

"She's in the hospital but will most likely be moved to another facility as soon as possible; Medicare won't let her stay once she's out of the critical care unit." All the questions that came immediately to mind seemed stupid, like was she OK, was she going to live, and so forth. I knew she wasn't OK and that it would probably be for the best if she did pass on; after all, what kind of life was she going to live now?

"How soon can I go see her?" I asked instead.

"Well you can go see her anytime, once we have her placed. But she's not going to recognize you," he added. "I went to visit her today, and she thought I was her brother, Fred. Then to add insult to injury, she told me to get the hell out of her room, that this was my entire fault." His voice was faltering now, and I could tell he was holding back tears.

"The Mrs. and I have taken care of her these past six years, and at our own expense, included her in our lives and home. We've made sacrifices, and now look at all the thanks we get," he said. I knew this was a tough emotional place for them to find themselves in, and I wanted to say something that would be at least somewhat comforting.

"It was very difficult when we had to place my mother in a nursing home," I said. "It's never easy, and my father felt guilty because he thought he should have been able to do something more for her."

"You know that the Mrs. promised my dad right before he died that she would never put Gertrude in one of those places," he said. "The Mrs. is going to be devastated about this. What am I going to tell her now?"

"Look," I said, "you don't have a choice anymore unless you can hire round-the-clock nursing care. Your wife can't possibly take care of her in this condition; we all know that." Actually, I felt that they should have placed her in a nursing center long ago. She had been going downhill for the last year. It's hard to accept that, though, when it's your own mother. I knew just how they felt.

"We will still need you to come and do art therapy with her. It's the only nice thing she has left now," he said. "You can still go see her, can't you?"

"Don't worry, Professor, I go into those places all the time. In fact, I'm at the hospital right now. When you know where she's going to be, just give me a call. I'll find her," I said.

"I want to thank you for all you've done for my mother over the years — and for us," he added.

"You are definitely welcome, and don't worry. I'll be there," I said.

"She just wants to come home," the Professor said.

"I know, that's what everybody wants, but don't worry: I promise I'll be there for her," I said.

"Thank you again. I'll call you as soon as we know what we're going to do." We said good-bye at that point, and I hung up the phone. But I kept thinking about Gertrude and what might lie ahead for her and her family. I remembered when my own mother had to go into a nursing facility; every time I visited she cried and clung to me, begging me to stay, to take her home. But first let me back up and tell this story when it really begins: when I met Gertrude.

Chapter 3

October 28, 1999

The first time I met Gertrude, she was only 88 years old, living with her son and his family in the nicest part of town. The street was lined with elms that had withstood the blight of the 1950s and '60s. Dappled light shone down through their graceful limbs in the warm months and cast elegant shadows in the winter. The surface of the village pond was adrift with ducks and duck babies, while along its borders gathered mothers with human babies.

Gertrude's family lived in a looming stone house, set high on a hill. Many steps led up to the front door. At first it reminded me of a castle because it was covered with vines. Azaleas and other classic perennials grew along its borders. For all I knew, they'd been planted when the house was built, in 1926. Even today, as I walk up the steps, I always remember the wonderful dampness and green smells that greeted me that first day, before I went inside and met Gertrude's family.

I spoke with the Professor and his wife in their living room, mostly about my credentials, work experience, and fee schedule. They told me that their mother had been living with them since her husband died and that she had become severely depressed. The visiting nurse had advised them to find an art or music therapist to work with Gertrude. Antidepressants had failed to lift her spirits. After some conversation, we all agreed that I should give it a go with her. Truth be told, they had probably run out of other options.

"Do you think you can help my mother?" the Professor asked.

"I'll certainly give it my best, sir," I said.

"Fine, fine," he said. "Shall we go upstairs and meet her then?"

"Oh yes, sir, I would love to do that, but it is getting rather late. Why don't we schedule a meeting soon? I suggested.

Gertrude lived on the second floor. Her bedroom was over the garage, so it was hot in the summer and cold in the winter. Her only window looked out into the alley behind the house. Her companions in the alley were the neighborhood cats, dogs, and squirrels on a regular basis, or the city garbage truck on Mondays and Thursdays.

Breakfast, lunch, and dinner were delivered to Gertrude's room on a tray.

She had the same breakfast *and* lunch every day, the entire time I worked for the Professor and his wife — at least the days I was there. Of course it was not like that all the time. On special holidays and birthdays her family helped her downstairs, and she ate with them in the dining room.

Every once in a while I would meet with Gertrude's family to review her well-being and whatever progress we had made. The meetings were difficult to schedule with them. The Mrs. volunteered a lot at the museum and the Professor was a research scientist who frequently traveled all around the world. They were always busy. They were also trying to do what they thought was the right thing for their mother — keeping her at home. God bless them for trying.

A maid cleaned the house, a visiting nurse specialist checked her vital signs, and an aide came every other day to bathe and dress her. I came on Mondays and Thursdays for an hour to do the activities. But she remained depressed and they couldn't understand *why*. So we continued to have these meetings. I would tell them that Gertrude needed more stimulation and interaction, and they would tell me that I made a difference in her life.

"You have absolutely extended my mother's life," the Professor told me. "Thank you from the bottom of my heart!"

November 24, 1999

Gertrude has told me her whole life story in bits and pieces over the years. Because she repeats herself all the time, I have gradually memorized every detail. When I went back to meet Gertrude, her son, the Professor, took me upstairs and then down a long, dark hallway to her room. He knocked gently at the door before entering. The room was dark like the hall that led up to it. It was a small room, filled with big furniture. Along one wall was a couch piled with stacks of laundry. Two chests were set on different walls; one had a mirror at the top, and the other a big television set. The television was on, but Gertrude wasn't watching. She was sitting at a card table sorting photographs into piles.

Her son spoke tentatively. "Mother, I have someone here I'd like you to meet."

When she didn't look up, he tried again, louder this time. "Mother, someone is here to visit with you today." Gertrude looked up from her photographs.

"What did you say?"

"I have the art teacher with me, and she wants to meet you."

"I don't paint anymore, can't see right. Now get out of here." Gertrude turned back to her photographs as if that were the end of it. I shrugged. Now what? He tried again. "Mother, the art teacher is right here, and she ...." But Gertrude cut him off in mid-sentence.

"I'm *not* painting, I'm old!"

His pager started beeping. He turned to me with relief.

"I'll just let you two get to know each other then. Good luck." Then he was out the door, and I stood facing her alone.

"Hi. I guess you already know that I'm an artist," I said. "May I sit down?"

She looked directly at me and said, "Suit yourself, but I'm not painting today. I'm sorting through my things."

"Why don't you let me help?" I asked. I glanced around and found a straight-backed chair to pull over to the table.

"This is about all I've got left of my memories," she said, without looking up. "They don't let me have any of my own furniture since I'm in such cramped quarters. After my husband died, they came and got me, and I've been stuck in this room ever since." She sighed and shook her head.

"How long have you been here, Gertrude?" I asked.

"I just told you — since my husband died." And with that, she sat back and jutted her jaw at me.

"I was thinking in terms of days and months," I said.

"Eight months, more or less," she replied. "Why do you care anyway? You don't even know me."

Initial meetings have always been difficult for me. What does one say to a person who is having a healthy response to tough circumstances? "Hello, I'm going to make this all better for you?"

Instead, I leaned closer to her, our faces almost touching. "Your family thought you might like to start some art lessons," I said. "I'm your entertainment, so to speak."

"I used to paint with the nuns," she said. "It was a long time ago." Then she pushed her wheelchair back and reached over toward an old dresser. She began pulling out the many drawers and examining the contents in several of them. Finally she found what she was looking for.

"Ah-ha! This is the first painting I ever did! The nuns used to say to me, 'Just paint what you see, Gertrude. Just paint what you see!' " She sat back and smiled broadly. In her lap she held a painting: an autumn landscape on a small canvas board. So she *had* painted before.

"That's nice," I said. But I was more interested in the dresser behind her. Whatever was in it, the contents of all those drawers?

For some reason, she reminded me of my grandmother. When Gertrude opened the drawers, I had glimpsed bright materials, maybe buttons, letters, and underwear all mixed up together, little compartments representing the different directions her life had taken. "My goodness," I said, "it's your mother's dresser."

"No it's not. It's my cupboard," she replied.

"It looks like an old dresser to me," I said.

Gertrude scowled at me from her wheelchair. "Now just why is it that you are here?" she asked.

"I'll be coming back on Monday to teach you how to paint," I said.

She frowned again. "I just got through showing you. I already know how to paint!"

"Yes, I know, Gertrude, but I'll be seeing you again next Monday."

Then I was out the door, back down the dark hall, and the flight of stairs. I didn't feel like taking up any more time, so I slipped out the back door, got in my car, and began the long drive home. Gertrude's family and I had already agreed upon a contractual arrangement for the next six months. It was good money. I needed the money, and I thought Gertrude needed something to do.

If it hadn't been such an easy thing to get out of though, I really don't think I could have considered working with her at first. She certainly wasn't very friendly for one thing and for another, what does someone say to a person who is suffering?"

There is only one thing you can say and it is this: "you **are** going to get better!"

Chapter 4

November 24, 1999

Fall had finally arrived, and the weather had been crisp during the day, but this particular evening it had begun to drizzle and it seemed darker than usual for the ride home. I was later than normal getting into traffic because of the interview with Gertrude, so by the time I got on the beltway that goes around the city, a bottleneck of traffic had formed, cars and big trucks all trying to squeeze into two lanes going north.

I had just moved to an old, rambling farmhouse about 30 minutes out of town. It was in the country, a place that was more of a hamlet than a town. The house stood at the intersection of two roads. It was nearly 200 years old and in earlier days had served as an inn for travelers on their way to Baltimore. At some point in the house's life, someone had remodeled, and now nothing was historically accurate.

My landlady had purchased the place at a foreclosure auction two years earlier. There was still an old livery stable in great disrepair on the front end of the property, but that was the only building that remained as it had been from the earlier part of the century.

Her hope was to save enough money to have the stable torn down before it fell down. The house and the yard were a bit overgrown and run-down, but it was my idea of semi-retirement to the country, where I could relax and do some landscape painting in the relative peace and quiet, far from the madding crowd.

So, the drive was longer than if I had remained in the suburbs, but I was getting used to it. I turned on the radio to listen to the news and get the weather report. It was nearly Thanksgiving. Outside my car window the drizzle was starting to transform into slushy rain mixed with snow. It was getting harder to see the road as I approached another part of the highway where several more lanes of traffic would be merging.

The traffic was barely moving now, and cars were inching forward, creeping along at about 10 miles an hour. My lane had come to a full stop, so I fiddled with the radio dials, waiting. All of a sudden, I felt the rear end of my car rise, as if lifted by some unseen and alien force.

"*What's happening?*" I worried. I turned to look out my window and what I saw took my breath away: I was looking directly into the lettering on a door of a large freight truck. At the same time, the end of my car was being lifted off the road.

I finally found my voice. "What *is* happening?" I cried out.

The truck must have come too close to my little sports car. The lug nuts from the truck wheels had gotten stuck under the wheel well of my car. When the truck's wheels went forward, my car was jacked up. Worse yet, the driver of the truck probably hadn't even seen me and my little car because of the darkness. I had to take desperate action or be crushed under the wheels of the tractor trailer.

I shifted into first gear and stepped on the gas, hoping to break away. I gave it more gas, and the car wiggled from side to side for a moment. My heart was in my throat, I knew this because I could feel it throbbing there. I shifted again into second gear and once more slammed my foot on the gas.

It was then that I heard a loud ripping sound, smelled burned rubber, and felt the car drop down to the roadway and bump forward. Traffic had started to move again, too, and the trucker, oblivious to me, was rolling away down the road. I didn't dare stop to evaluate the damage, because the traffic was moving faster now, and I was afraid I'd be killed on the side of the road if I stopped. I drove all the way home like that, with a sense of apprehension. I just couldn't shake it.

When I pulled up in the driveway, the back porch lights came on, and my landlady stood waiting for me to get out of my car, but the look on her face told me everything.

I slowly climbed out of the car and turned around for my own look. The entire back panel had been ripped off, and the bumper was hanging down to the ground on the driver's side.

"I'm just a wreck!" was what I said to her. I was trying to be funny.

"Oh my God!" she said. "Let me give you a big hug!"

I held my hand up, keeping her at arm's length. "I don't want a big hug. I need a drink!"

So we went inside where it was warm. I moved toward the fire in the fireplace. "I heated up some of the vegetable soup," she said. "Would you like some?"

"Do I have to get it myself?" I asked. She didn't say anything, so I had a moment to think about what I did want. "Never mind," I said to her. "I'm going to make that drink instead."

I went downstairs to the kitchen. The old house had been built into a hill, and since it had once served as an inn, the kitchen and the washroom were on a lower level, along with a couple of bedrooms. She lived downstairs and I lived upstairs.

She had a kitchen, and I had a room with a view. Tonight though, I felt as if I were trespassing into her domain. I felt out of place in there, looking through her cabinets for a bottle of bourbon. I finally found it, hidden behind a pile of Tupperware containers that had fallen down inside the cupboard.

It was like looking through the contents of someone's personal things after they have died. I knew that the Tupperware had come from a time when she had been married. She didn't work then; she stayed home, hung drapes, and cooked delicious dinners for her husband. Now, all the stuff she had accumulated during her marriage was either packed in boxes in the attic or stuffed into the cupboards in the kitchen. She had hung on to the house by renting out rooms to transient people, roommates all, never relationships that lasted for very long.

It was sad to be standing in the kitchen, holding onto a bottle of liquor and knowing there was a warm fire upstairs and the comfort of a friend waiting for me. But I couldn't get into it, so I didn't go upstairs. I remained alone, drinking straight from the bottle. Standing there in her kitchen was like standing in the middle of someone else's life, where every moment had been put away forever, out of sight, into the cupboards. I had cleaned out my own apartment before moving into this house with her. I had hired an estate sales person, who packed up almost everything I owned and auctioned it all off. I took my check for $2,000 dollars and moved into Evelyn's house with my clothes, art supplies, computer, and some paintings.

I was depressed all of a sudden. Heck, when I really thought about it, I was much worse off than even old Gertrude. She at least had hung on to her memories by placing everything meaningful in her cupboard, but I had thrown mine away. Now my car was trashed, too. I wasn't even certain I could drive to work — or anywhere for that matter. With that realization, I sat down on the cold stone floor of Evelyn's kitchen and cried.

I woke up the next morning with the sound of light rain against my window. I could hear some birds chirping, though, and the sound of music from a lower floor of the house. I had taken too many drinks the night before but had somehow managed to climb the three flights of stairs to my room and dropped onto the top of my bed before passing out. I hadn't gotten under the covers either, so I was still dressed in the same clothes that I had worn to work the day before. My head was throbbing, and I was thirsty.

It was like coming out of a bad dream. I tried to figure out what time it was and to remember what had happened. Then I remembered my car. "Darn!" It was the day before Thanksgiving. I wondered if I could even get in touch with my insurance agent, much less get a rental car. I looked around for my watch. The estate liquidator had accidentally sold my alarm clock, and I hadn't replaced it yet.

I figured it must be going on noon. With this thought, I bolted straight out of bed and ran down the hall to the top of the stairs. I called out, "What time is it?"

Evelyn shouted back, "Eleven-thirty!"

"I might need to borrow your car!" I yelled, and then moved to the top of the stairs so I wouldn't have to keep raising my voice. My head hurt. Suddenly Evelyn was standing in my field of vision.

"When do you need it?" she asked. "I've got to pick up Mickey at noon from his school."

She was standing at the bottom of the stairs that led up to the third floor in an old pink terry cloth robe, holding a cup of coffee in one hand and a cigarette in the other. Mickey was her 11-year-old son, who went to a private Christian school somewhere in the county. His real name was Michael Bennett Skinner, III, but Evelyn had gotten into the habit of calling him Mickey when he was a baby.

"If I leave now, I can be back here by one-thirty," she said.

"I need to pick up Gray at the airport by three," I said. "Will I have enough time to get to the airport?"

"Oh gosh, yes!" she replied.

"You're not going to drive to the school dressed like that, are you?" I asked.

"Like *what*?"

"In that bathrobe," I said. Wasn't it obvious to her?

"Looked into the mirror yourself lately?" she asked. And with that remark, she tapped the long ash of her cigarette into the pot of a very dried-up plant that had died in a corner near the bottom of the stairs. Sometimes she could be really disgusting. I even thought she did it to me on purpose once in a while.

Then she disappeared into her room, and I could hear her moving things around. A couple of minutes later, she was bounding down the side stairs. I heard the slam of the back door and her car starting up, then the crunch of gravel.

I walked back down the hallway to my bathroom and looked into the mirror. It had probably been installed sometime in the 1930s. There were places around the edges where the silver on the back had been scratched off, and so it didn't reflect anything there. Consequently, parts of my hairline were missing at the top of the mirror. A flaw ran from top to bottom, causing a wavelike imperfection down the middle. I looked like a bad photo taken with a wide-angle lens. I looked like hell. The dark circles under my eyes were darker than usual, and my hair was bushy.

I looked out the bathroom window into the driveway behind the house. There was my little sports car, with one side hanging, nearly ripped off the frame. In comparison, I thought, I looked worse than the car. I was going to have to take a shower — that was all there was to it. After all, the show must go on. My son was expecting me to pick him up at the airport latter that afternoon.

After about 30 minutes, I'd had my shower, dressed, and was drinking coffee, waiting for Evelyn to return and the insurance people to call me back. The insurance company called first. They had it all figured out. I would drop my car off at the body shop for an estimate, and the rental car people would meet me there. But best of all, I got to arrange all the details around my trip to the airport. The other good news: Now I wouldn't have to wait around for Evelyn to show up, because I didn't need to borrow her car. Suddenly I felt relieved. I wasn't at the mercy of anything now! That feeling was not to last. My phone rang, and I assumed it would be the car rental place calling to confirm. I yawned and picked up the receiver.

"Hello."

"This is John," I heard.

I was surprised to hear his deep baritone voice. We hadn't talked in nearly six months, not since Ben and Debbie had married. Trouble ? Why else would he call? John is my sons' father. Gray must have missed his plane. The younger of our sons, he lived with John in San Antonio. He was supposed to be flying

over Tennessee on a Southwest flight right now, eating peanuts.
"Gray's flight isn't delayed is it?" I asked. There was a long pause and then his voice again, now not so melodious or resonant.
"No, that's not why I called."
"What's up?" I asked.
"Ben's tried to kill himself," was what he said. I was certain I hadn't heard him correctly.
"What did you say, John? I couldn't hear you very well, radio's turned on." I reached over to turn the radio off so that I could hear.
"I *said* that Ben tried to take his *life* yesterday afternoon," he said.

I sat down on the floor. It felt like the air had gone out of me. At the same time, I couldn't feel any emotion, either. It was a strange sensation. I can only compare it to an anxiety attack when there is a terrible lack of air, the feeling of suffocation, but not because someone is strangling you. There I was sitting on the floor of my room, looking under my bed, where the dust balls hadn't had time to form yet.

I had just learned that my son had tried to leave this world behind. It was sad and it was strange to learn all this. I felt as if I were hearing about someone else's life, not my son's life. I shuddered and remembered the last time we all were together.

I looked at my watch. I had to leave for the airport soon. Now I felt another wave of urgency. I had to somehow handle what seemed like a hundred things before driving home in rush-hour traffic in an unfamiliar car, possibly in the dark. And my dear son had tried to take his life.

June 10, 1999

I remembered when he was happy. Ben had met Debbie several months earlier at a restaurant where they both worked. He was a chef, and she managed the front. They had dated briefly — nothing serious, it seemed at the time. One day he hadn't shown up for work, and Debbie had gone to look for him. After quite a long hunt, she found Ben beneath his bed. He seemed to be unconscious, but in fact he was having a grand mal seizure. He had been missing for 24 hours, but no one knew how long he had been under the bed. Debbie called 911, and Ben was rushed to the hospital.

None of the many exams was conclusive. But five little bleeds in his brain had showed up on a CAT scan. Because of my mother's impaired neurology, it was suggested he go in for more extensive testing at Johns Hopkins. I was standing in his room at the hospital, deciding how to transport Ben over to Hopkins, when Debbie walked in. She looked even more nervous than the situation called for and said that she had something important to tell us. We stopped talking for a moment to listen.

"I'm pregnant," was what she said.

He never made it to Hopkins. Instead, in spite of my protests, he sold his car and bought Debbie an engagement ring. She wanted to be near her family when the baby came, so they drove to Florida in her Toyota near the end of February.

I flew to Naples, Florida, with my best friend, Elliot, in mid-June for the wedding. The service took place in a fancy hotel down by the sea, and the bride's family had decorated extravagantly. The wedding pictures were taken at dusk; the sky was peach and lavender, and the wedding party was beautiful there on the beach with the wind blowing gently and the sunset behind them. I didn't know anyone at the wedding except for my two sons, Elliot, and my ex-husband, John.

The photographer took a long time on the beach. When we finally went back to the reception, it had grown dark. I think I was probably the only person there with two escorts, Elliot and John. As it turned out, we were all seated at the same table; next to us were Debbie's parents, grandparents, and a couple of siblings who weren't sitting at the head table with the rest of the wedding party.

"This is cozy," Elliot said once we were seated, but before I had a chance to respond, John interrupted.

"Hey, if you two aren't going to drink, can I have your drink tickets?" he asked.

"Sure," I said, "knock yourself out." Elliot and I both handed over two tickets each, and John took off for the bar. "Some things never change," I said. Elliot laughed and nodded in agreement.

The night wore on. Along with the DJ, Debbie's family had hired one of her cousins, an Elvis impersonator, to sing as part of the entertainment. He walked around with a wireless microphone singing love songs, interrupted only by Ben, who was saying all kinds of romantic things. "This is the happiest day of my whole life," he said, and continued proclaiming his love for Debbie.

John must have managed to acquire other drink tickets, too, because there were about seven empty glasses in front of his seat when I checked to see about him. Before too long, I spotted him coming our way with two more drinks, one in each hand. He managed to negotiate the dance floor without spilling anything and dropped down in the chair next to me, grinning from ear to ear.

"Hey, you probably should slow down, cowboy," I said to him.

"Hell, it's our son's wedding. I'll drink as much as I want," he said. Then he leaned closer and put his arm around the back of my chair. "This is some kind of circus, isn't it?" he asked.

"I must admit that Elvis is certainly a special touch," I said. He leaned; grabbing the table for more support, then spoke again, only louder this time.

"If you and I had done this thing, we'd have done it right. Look at this shit, will you?" He reached toward the centerpiece, grabbed the bottom of the vase, and pulled it toward us. The tablecloth came with it and some of the dishes. "Look at this!" he said. John held up the vase for me to get a better look. "It looks like some kind of damned funeral urn," he said. He was right about that. It was a smaller replica of the kind of urn one might see in a cemetery except that it was painted silver and had fake ferns growing out of the top. Elvis had waltzed over to our table right about then, and he asked Elliot what he would like to hear him sing.

"Who the hell is that?" John asked me, and both of us started laughing. I realize now that my laughter must have encouraged him, because the next thing he said got both of us kicked out of the reception.

He sat back in his chair. First he looked almost angelic, then devilish. His arms were crossed in front of him, and he was shaking with mirth.

He said "Honey, these people aren't Eye-talian, they're just cheap Jew bastards!"

And this was supposed to be the happiest day of Ben's life.

November 24, 1999

I was still holding onto the phone. "John, are you still there?" I asked.

"I don't know much about what happened," was all he said. "But I just wanted to tell you before Gray gets there."

"I don't know what to say," I said.

"Well, I'm sorry," he said. There was another pause between us. "It's really hard to know what to tell you. I don't have any details except that Debbie called me this morning."

"Is he in the hospital and can I talk to him?" I asked.

"She didn't give me that information, but I'll try to find out and get back with you," he said. "I've got to go now though, we'll talk later." That was the end of our conversation because he hung up before I could get another word in.

I felt paralyzed there on the floor. I could still hear birds outside the window; they seemed to be my only company. The sky had begun to turn gray, and the rain was really starting to come down, mirroring my mood. I kept hearing one phrase going on inside my head, only it was more like a prayer, and it was this: *Please God help me.* I looked out the window and saw that the sky was now obscured by clouds. Large droplets of rain were starting to fall again on the porch roof. It was as if nature was crying for me because I couldn't. I wondered then if God really knew what was going on in my life at all or if I were really as insignificant as I felt right then.

I could hear the gravel on the driveway crunching and realized that Evelyn and Mickey must be home. The back door slammed, and I could hear them bringing stuff into the house. She was irritated at him again. I didn't hear what she was saying, but I could tell by her tone that he was in trouble. The poor kid spent most of his free time in his room downstairs, grounded for stupid infractions like not putting dishes in the dishwasher correctly or forgetting to fold her wash. It was always one thing or another.

I had started down the stairs when I heard her tell Mickey to go to his room. "Michael, go straight to your room and don't come out again until all the clothes on the floor are folded," she said. They were standing in the living room, and his head was hanging down. He seemed to be inspecting the carpet. His book bag was dangling from his right arm, forming a lumpy pile on the carpet, and in the other hand he held a wrinkled brown jacket. He looked more like an old hobo than an 11-year-old boy.

"Get *downstairs*," she screamed. Then she turned to me and, with a flick of her head, gestured me to follow. "Let's go," she commanded, and then she was out the door without looking to see if I had followed. I didn't have a chance to tell her I wouldn't need the ride after all. I followed her out to the driveway to explain this. She was standing next to my car, lighting up another cigarette. As I approached, she blew a long stream of smoke toward the car. I remember being amazed by this, because any other mere human being wouldn't have been able to light the cigarette in the first place with all the rain coming down.

"I won't need a ride. I got in touch with the insurance agent, and it's all handled," I said. She looked at me in disbelief and then took another long drag off her cigarette.

"Do you mean I came all the way back here and you don't need the car?"

"Yeah, I was able to get the logistics sorted out. I'm going to drive to the body shop, and the car rental people will meet me there." Her lip curled at this, and she threw the cigarette down on the ground. It landed near my feet and sizzled as the rain hit the burning end. I took a step back and considered what to tell her next. I wasn't so sure she would want to hear the rest of the story.

"Look, I'm sorry you went out of your way for me. I appreciate it, I really do."

"Oh that's OK," she replied. "Everybody else takes advantage of my good nature — what makes you any different?"

"I'm not trying to take advantage of you, Evelyn," I said. "It's been a rough morning, and I got some more bad news, so it's all been kind of complex and confusing and Ben-is-in-the-hospital!" The last part of the sentence just seemed to rush out of me. I hadn't intended on telling anyone just yet, much less my newly acquired landlady.

"What do you mean he's in the hospital?" Her surly look had transformed into one of condescension. She crossed her arms against her chest now as she waited for my response. The rain was still coming down, and it was turning colder. I rubbed my hands together before holding them out in front of me, like a protective shield. With my palms up, I faced her in the driveway, as if blocking her. I felt defensive and very alive.

"He tried to kill himself. I don't know any more details than that," I blurted out. "If his father calls, can you take a message for me until I get back?"

The look on her face changed to one of surprise. She strode across the drive until she was so close to me I could smell the smoke on her breath. She wrapped her arms around me in a big hug. I felt smothered, and the cigarette smell was nauseating. I stood awkwardly in her embrace with an intense desire to leave immediately. I wanted to be released from the stronghold of her arms. She made me nervous.

"Let me go," I said. "I've got to get to the airport." She let me go and I went straight to my car. Despite the outward condition, the car started right up. I knew I would make it to the body shop in one piece. As I backed down the driveway, I rolled down the window and yelled out to her. For some reason or another, I felt sorry for her.

What I called back to her that day was what I told all of my patients, no matter what was going on: "Don't worry; it's all going to be OK." Then I waved good-bye and drove down the road.

Chapter 5

November 25, 1999

Thanksgiving was clear and bright. The sky was a brilliant blue, and I could see the entire valley from the third floor of the house. It looked washed clean from the rain we'd had the day before. My car was safe in the body shop, and my younger son was still sleeping in my room. I had camped out on the floor of my studio where I had a coffee machine and a small refrigerator. This convenience made it possible to have breakfast without going downstairs and risking waking anyone up. I had just started on my second cup of coffee when the phone rang. I jumped up to get it before the second ring.

This time it was Debbie, my son's wife. "Hi, I guess you heard what happened," she said. "Ben is in the hospital here, and I thought I should call because he doesn't have phone privileges yet."

I was wondering why she hadn't called me earlier, but I held my tongue. Instead I asked, "Is Ben OK?"

"Oh yes, he was just under stress. I don't think he was sleeping much because he was getting up to feed the baby a couple times a night, and he works a lot at the restaurant," she replied. "But the baby's fine, though."

She had just given birth to their first child, a boy, only a month before, and I felt sorry for her having to carry so much responsibility. "It must be very difficult for you right now," I said. I knew that she didn't like me very much, especially after the incident with John at their wedding. I was hoping to use the conversation to bring us closer together. She started to cry. "You don't have any idea how hard things have been!" she said. "He's been impossible these last weeks."

"Do you mean the baby or Ben?" I asked.

"Ben, of course!" She was almost screaming into the phone now. I held the phone away from my ear and tried to imagine her standing in a phone booth in the hospital corridor, separated from her husband who was probably down the hall in the psychiatric unit. I looked out my window. I could see that the sky was a beautiful hue, the fields and hills begging to be painted. I desperately wanted to be outside in that landscape of hills when I realized that Debbie was still talking to me.

"He was working all the time, and I thought he should at least help me with the baby a little bit, so he was doing the night feedings," she said. Then she started to sob again. "It's not fair, it's just not fair!" she cried.

"What's not fair, dear?" I asked.

"I can't believe he did this to me!" she said. At this point in our conversation I wasn't quite sure how to respond and still find out how my son really was without sounding unsympathetic toward her.

"I'm sorry you've had to go through so much," I said. "It must be terrible, but can you tell me when can I speak with Ben?"

"I'll tell him to call you after his evaluation," she said. I could hear a great deal of commotion in the background now, and then the receiver went dead and she was gone.

Now I was faced with the situation that I hate the most: not knowing. I decided to sit around by the phone anyway, hoping that sooner or later he would call me. Then I would relax, I told myself.

The phone rang a few more times that morning, but it was various friends calling to find out about Ben. I didn't have anything more to tell them, so our conversations were short. Most of them had family dinners or parties to attend anyway. I had already decided to take Gray out for Thanksgiving dinner for two reasons: It gave us something to do, and I hoped it would prevent me from feeling weird and lost on another holiday. I hated holidays now. My sons were the only two family members I had left in the whole world, now that my mother was locked up in the home. I still had a brother, sister, and father, but none of us had talked for a long time. They were as lost to me as if they had died. We hadn't had a fight or anything; it just seemed as if we'd all lost interest over the years.

Thanksgiving vacation passed slowly. Gray and I took long walks and waited by the phone. As I look back, I see that I was numb during that time. It was almost like watching a movie.

"Why do you think he did it, Mom?" Gray asked.

"Maybe the pain of being alive was too much for him," I answered. "I don't know, I always thought he was happy."

Finally Ben did call, but he had kept us waiting so long that I had become anxious and afraid by then; I felt as if my heart were going to break open. Gray and I hovered over the phone together to hear what he was saying. The hospital had done some tests, he told us. They had found something in his brain they thought had contributed to the seizures.

"What kind of seizures?" I asked.

"I was having some kind of strange daydream," he explained. "The devil was speaking to me from the mirror in my bedroom. It's happened before, but when I started to get up at night, I would see him there all the time. Then I started to see him at work, and he was talking to me, telling me stuff."

"What did he tell you?" I asked.

"Well, he told me to hurt the baby. He told me I should suffocate the baby and that I should . . ." He stopped talking and started to sob. "I'm so sorry," he said, "I didn't mean it, I didn't. I told the doctor that I don't think I did anything to hurt him."

"I'm sure you didn't do anything like that," I told him.

"Listen, I've got to go, Mom, they only allow me so long to

use the phone. I'll call you tomorrow. I think they're going to keep me here for a while."

"I love you," I said.

"Me too," he said. And then we hung up. I still couldn't cry, though. I thought I should have. I remember thinking how strange it all was that I couldn't feel any of the pain the others were feeling.

The days following the holiday were so beautiful. The wind had blown what was left of the fall leaves from the driveway and the lawn. Our house had been built into a great hill and the expansive lawn was a vibrant green. A series of flagstone steps curved up through the gardens in front, and flagstone terraces had been built across the lawn, probably to keep the hill from washing away.

Gray had decided to watch a football game on TV and had settled into a big leather chair in the den, leaving me to cast about for something to do. I stared down at the lawn, watching how the last of the leaves were being caught in the dead plants that remained in the garden. The wind had made them come alive, moving them about in the branches of the azaleas. Meanwhile I had a good view of the road that went by the house. Cars were whizzing south along the old route into the city of Baltimore. I wondered what the people in the cars would be doing when they got to wherever it was they were going. I felt alone and lost again.

Finally I decided it was too beautiful to remain inside on a day like this, especially after all the rain. Another walk would do me some good. I found my leather jacket and an old hat, and I pulled my hiking boots on, ready to go on a long jaunt. I reminded myself that this was why I had moved into the country in the first place, and besides, walking was a good way to alleviate depression. I put on my sunglasses and headed out the door into the back driveway. I heard a crunch of tires on the loose gravel before I saw the old station wagon pulling up. In fact, I nearly walked into the car because my eyes hadn't adjusted to the light yet. I was a little blind from the sun, but I did recognize the car.

It turned out to be my neighbor, Lewis, who lived up the road not far from us. He often came to visit, unannounced, and I gave a long sigh. I was never glad to see him. For some reason he liked to bring us strange-shaped stones and pieces of wood that he found around the reservoir. He would tell Evelyn and me that we could use all these interesting things as decoration in the gardens. Actually, I used the wood for kindling in the fireplace. Evelyn had carefully placed the stones along the driveway in the back as a kind of barrier, keeping people from parking their cars on the lawn.

Evelyn and I had lots of visitors that fall, and for some reason, when they drove up the back driveway, they always parked on the lawn. I found out later that we had become a kind of roadside attraction for all the single males who lived in the surrounding countryside. Evelyn and I were known as the two artists who lived in the old inn up on the hill. Lewis was no exception, only he came around nearly every day.

The old station wagon pulled to an abrupt halt on the gravel. I pushed my sunglasses back on my head so that I could see better. Lewis remained in the car, rolling the window down. "Hi, how'd you like some company?" he asked.

Actually I really didn't want company, and the last thing I needed was Lewis tagging along on my walk. I tried to think of a good reason to send him packing when I realized that there was someone else in the car with him. The other person leaned forward now, making it possible to see them both at once. Lewis's passenger was smiling at me. I moved toward the car, not sure now whether to send them on their way or to invite them inside.

"This is my friend Richard," Lewis said. I didn't say anything, just held up my hand in a universal greeting. Lewis must have sensed my reluctance to invite them in, because he continued talking. "We've been out all morning on a hike and thought you'd like the firewood we gathered," he said. I crossed my arms in front of my chest. What I didn't need was any more firewood from Lewis.

"Gee whiz, Lewis, we're in pretty good shape with wood right now. Evelyn's friend Tommy just brought us a load last week," I said. I turned and pointed to the side of the house where a lumpy pile of wood lay where Tommy had dumped it. I crossed my arms again and stood there waiting for Lewis to get the hint and leave.

Instead, his friend Richard was opening the door and climbing out of the car. He spoke for the first time. "Then I'll be helping you stack that wood," he said. Not even waiting for a reply, he walked directly across the drive to the pile of wood and then turned around. Richard was looking intensely at me, and I shifted nervously. "That's supposing it's OK with you if I stack your wood," he said. He was still smiling.

He had certainly taken me by surprise. "Actions speak louder than words," I finally replied. But I was charmed by his boldness and by the practicality of his suggestion. I took a step in his direction; something about him was intriguing.

"Is Evelyn home?" Lewis asked.

I had forgotten Lewis. I turned back and saw that Lewis was still sitting in the car. "She's in New Jersey, won't be home till sometime this evening," I said. "Why don't you go inside and watch the football game with my son Gray?" Meanwhile Richard was already stacking the wood, paying no attention to me or Lewis. A man of action I thought, how refreshing. I found I was smiling, too; I felt uplifted for the first time in several days.

"Come on, Lewis, I'll show you where Gray is, and you can help yourself to whatever you want to eat," I said. We went into the house together.

"Got any beer?" he asked.

On Sunday I drove Gray back to the airport. We arrived early, and I decided to wait with him until the plane docked at the gate. All around us, groups of people were saying good-bye. Babies in strollers, young men in uniform, college kids with book bags, and grandmas and grandpas were embracing, kissing one another. In that respect, we were like the rest of the crowd. Gray was leaving, too.

It was then that I started to feel a pain in my chest. It swelled up and moved to my throat, one big lump. I couldn't swallow and I couldn't talk. It was as if all the things I wanted to say had never been said, and now they had formed a huge ball in my throat that remained stuck there. Gray patted me on the back. My suffering had arrived at the worst of times, here at the airport, in front of people I didn't even know.

"Are you OK?" he asked. It seemed as if that was the only question either of us had asked each other in the last several days. It was slightly humorous in a strange kind of way that only he and I could appreciate. I smiled at him.

"I'm not going to die, if that's what you mean," I said.

"He's going to be fine, Mom," Gray said. "The doctors will find out what's in his head and fix it."

"I don't trust doctors. The last time a Doctor told me everything was going to go well, we ended up sticking my mother in the home," I said. Then I started to cry, little sobs, my shoulders going up and down. Gray gave me another hug, and we ambled over to the gate where they had started to load the plane.

"I'll call you soon," he said. Then he turned into the line with the rest of the passengers. I watched until he had rounded the corner, and then he was gone. I was left standing there in a room full of people, some coming and some going, but I felt more alone than I had in my whole life.

I walked slowly out to my car. There was no reason for me to rush anywhere now. Nobody was waiting for me to come home; there was no boyfriend, no husband, no parents calling, and most of my friends were out of town. Evelyn had gone off again to spend time with her friends on the Eastern shore. Mickey was spending the holiday with his father. The house would be dark when I got there.

Chapter 6

December 6, 1999

Monday was a work day, and I was relieved that I would have something to do besides listen for the phone to ring. In fact, I had taken it off the hook the night before. I didn't think that I could process any more information. I was tired and I needed to sleep.

My first client to see that morning was Gertrude. I loved driving through the neighborhood where she and her family lived. I drove in what I call the long way, around the fish ponds and the fountains spraying water in the middle. Then I drove up the alley behind the houses, which was the best way to park, I wouldn't have to climb all the steps leading up to the front. I had figured this out on my first visit, that there was an entrance in the back of the house. The dog greeted me at the back door, jumping up and knocking everything I had been carrying out of my hands, onto the floor.

"Scout, stop jumping!" the Mrs. called. She came out of the kitchen, wiping her hands on a dishtowel. She was a pretty blonde, slightly overweight, and flushed from whatever she had been doing in the kitchen. "I'm so sorry," she said.

I wish people would stop saying that to me, I thought. "Oh that's all right!" I said. I felt clumsy standing there with jars of paint rolling all over the hallway. The Mrs. stooped over to help me pick everything up. Together we managed to fit all the paint jars back into the cardboard box I had been holding.

"Scout gets excited whenever anyone comes into the house," she explained.

"Just tell him to get off next time. Gertrude's all ready for you, she even remembered you'd be coming!" she said. She smiled brightly and then turned and went back to her household chores. Meanwhile I began the ascent of the stairs with Scout right behind me, sniffing my rear end. I knocked at Gertrude's door, but before she answered, Scout had crashed through and was bouncing up to where she was sitting. The room was completely dark, even though it was still morning. All the window shades had been pulled shut, and the lights were turned off.

"Good morning!" I cried. "Let's turn some lights on. I can hardly see you, and get those shades up!"

"I like it dark," she replied. "You may turn on the light by the table, but please leave the shades alone."

She wasn't dressed yet and was wearing only a nightdress. Her hair was pushed up into a little nightcap, with wisps sticking out around the edges. She was holding a rosary in her hands, and a black Bible was lying open on her lap. The table to which she referred was the same card table I had seen earlier. It had been moved over to the window with a little bit of light coming in. On top of the table was a tray with leftover food on it. I picked up the tray to move it, but there wasn't anywhere to place it that didn't already have something else on it. I sighed and looked around the room. "Look, I'm just going to take the tray downstairs," I said. When I came back into the kitchen though, the Mrs. was taking a pan of little cookies out of the oven. Other batches were already cooling on the tops of all the counters and the table. So, for the second time that day, I felt like the world's biggest klutz, standing there with the tray in my hands and no place to put it down.

"Oh, dear, I'm so sorry!" she said. "I'm in the middle of baking for the museum's art auction this afternoon. Just put it on the floor, will you?"

"What about the dog?" I asked.

"What about him?" She looked mystified at this.

"Won't he eat off the tray?"

"Oh it's perfectly OK, he eats off Gertrude's trays all the time," she said.

I left the tray where she directed and went upstairs again. This time Gertrude had moved her wheelchair over to the card table in front of the window. She was leaning over the table and looking out from underneath the shade.

"Gotta keep an eye on 'em," she explained.

"You have to keep an eye on whom?"

"There's some men been trying to get into my room. Why, they put their ladders up to my windows and try to get in," she said. "That's why I always pull down the shades!" She sat back in the chair, and her lower lip was sticking out the same way it had the day I had met her, so I knew better than to challenge her about the men, whoever they were.

I moved over to the table, sat down in the only chair in her room, and pulled the shade about halfway up the window. She grimaced at the light that was now streaming into her room, holding her hands over her eyes.

"Jesus, Mary, and Joseph!" she yelled.

I reached to put my hand on her shoulder. "Settle down. If we don't have light, we can't see to paint," I said.

"Will you pull it back down after we're done?" she asked.

"Of course I will, but we need to start painting now," I said. I had already spent enough time moving her tray downstairs, and I thought we ought to be getting on with it. I pulled a piece of watercolor paper off a tablet I had brought along and started to squirt tempera paint into her paint tray.

"I haven't painted for a long time," she said. "My hand hurts. I don't think I can do this today." She pulled a shawl that had been draped over the back of her wheelchair around her shoulders. "I'm cold," she added, as if for effect. So, I gave her the standard answer I give to everyone who has some kind of consideration about painting.

"That's wonderful," I said.

"What do you mean?" she asked, incredulously.

"I mean, I understand about your hand and the fact that you haven't painted for the last 50 years or so and that you're cold. Fact is, none of that stuff is going to prevent you from painting today with me! Here's what we're going to do," I said. I took her hand then and wrapped it around the paintbrush just as you would hold a pencil. And I started to paint with her, me holding her hand, and she following my movements. It wasn't too long before she was holding the brush on her own and filling in the lines I had drawn on the paper.

"This is OK," she said. "The first time I took painting lessons, it was with the nuns from our parish, only they took us out to a field and told the class to just paint what you see."

"That's wonderful," I responded.

"Is that your standard answer for everything?" she asked.

"No."

"Well you always seem to say it. What else do you tell people who paint with you?" she asked.

I thought a minute about that. I didn't want her to think that I did the same thing with everyone. I just wanted her to participate with me, to begin moving again. "Usually I say that it's good," I said.

"Hum, what other lies do you tell people in wheelchairs like me?"

"I'm not here to discuss other clients, Gertrude. Why don't you tell me something interesting about you instead?" I asked.

She stopped painting then and folded her hands in her lap. She looked at me for a long while before she spoke again. "I've got a secret," she said.

"What kind of secret?"

"You won't believe me, nobody does anymore."

"I'm fairly open-minded. Try me."

She paused for a moment, pulling a rosary out from the pocket in her housedress. She held it to her heart for a moment before speaking again.

"I pray for people. I pray for people and they get better, or their luck changes. When I was a kid, my grandfather used to bring all kinds of folks around when there was some kind of problem or something. Back then we didn't have the kind of medicine we have today."

I smiled. "So you would pray for these people, and their luck would change, is that it?" I asked. She shifted around in her wheelchair and looked me straight in the eye.

"You don't believe me either, do you?" she asked.

"Well, it is a little far-fetched," I said. "Heck, I don't think I've prayed for anything or anyone since I was a little kid. I'm not so sure there even is a God that knows about me and my personal problems anyway," I added.

"Do you have a problem, dear?" she asked.

"We all have problems, Gertrude," I said. "There's not a person on earth who doesn't have some kind of cross to bear. I mean, if you're alive, you've got issues." I hadn't planned on the discussion getting quite so personal on the first session together, and I felt somewhat uncomfortable about what she had just said. After all, she was just an old lady, with a touch of dementia.

She sighed. "Do you have something you need praying for?" she asked again.

"I don't discuss my personal life with my clients," I said.

"Give me a name." She reached into the pocket of her nightdress again and brought the rosary she had been holding earlier out in front of me for inspection. "I always pray, with this rosary, every day," she said.

"Don't be silly. That's just one of those plastic things you can get anywhere for a dollar," I informed her. Now I was the one to sit back in my chair, while we stared at one another. There was a long pause before she spoke.

"Suit yourself," she said. She put the rosary back into her pocket. "I guess that we'll just have to busy ourselves and paint. That's what you've come here to do with me, isn't it? These painting lessons are supposed to be a distraction from my otherwise-mundane existence. Be honest with me."

"Well, yes, that's exactly why your son and daughter-in-law have hired me," I confessed.

"They're *paying* you to do this?" She looked absolutely shocked, put the paintbrush down and pushed herself away from the card table with such force that her water glass spilled and ran down one leg of the table. "This is worse than charity, and what's more, I didn't ask for it!" I could tell that she was angry, so I didn't say anything. I just waited.

"I'm the only one left in my family who's not dead. My grandfather, parents, and even my brothers and sisters are all gone now," she said.

Gertrude pulled the shawl tighter around her, turned away from me as if she was ashamed that this was in fact the end of the road. There was another long silence. I wasn't sure that anything I could say would make a difference now, so I waited. I was hoping something would pop into my head, and then I had an idea.

"How would you like a new friend?" I asked.

"Do I have a choice?" she asked.

"Not really. Your son has contracted with me for the next six months, so you're kind of stuck with me, I guess. I'm supposed to come here twice a week, Mondays and Thursdays. You can tell me all about your life — and we'll paint, of course," I added quickly.

Gertrude smiled faintly now. "Why not? God knows I'm not going anywhere. *But* if I don't end up liking you, you're not continuing. Have we got a deal?"

"I believe you have a new friend," I said. We shook hands. "I'll be back on Thursday, and we'll try some more painting. Is that OK?"

"We'll see," she said. "Now get out of here and take that dog with you!"

It was the first week of December, and some of the stores and shops I passed had already put up Christmas decorations. A Salvation Army Santa Claus was ringing a bell outside of the Wal-Mart store where I got most of my art supplies. I looked down at the ground as I passed the alias Santa, because I had only a couple of dollars on me, and I needed them more than Santa did. Once inside the store I was bombarded by a Christmas extravaganza; boxes of lights were piled up in the front, and a whole section of the flower department had been converted over into a labyrinth of Christmas trees in all sizes, mechanical angels, and tinsel. I managed to find a large bottle of white tempera paint in the midst of all the decorations and got out of Wal-Mart without buying anything else — not even a single bulb.

My next stop was a private nursing home on Falls Road. I worked with an Alzheimer's unit there on Monday afternoons. I unpacked the art supplies from my car and piled them onto my carrying cart, wheeling the whole load into the long-term care facility. I had just signed in at the front desk when I was met by the activities director. She surprised me. "Why are you here?" she asked me.

"This is the day that I am scheduled to work here, you know that," I replied.

She put her hands on her hips then and looked me up and down. "Frankly, I thought you'd be on a plane headed for Florida by now," she said.

I really wasn't in any mood to discuss my son that morning. I had done nothing but answer people's questions about the whole situation for a week now. "Drop it, Anne," I said. "He's going to be OK, and it's all under control. He's still in the hospital."

"If it were my kid, I would have been on a plane by now," she said.

"You're making me late for the group, and besides, it's not your kid," I said.

"Have it your way!" Anne threw her hands up over her head and proceeded down the hallway in front of me. "I just don't understand you, that's all."

"Well, I'm easy to understand," I said. "I work because I need the money!"

The double doors to the special-care unit loomed in front

of us. Anne reached them first and punched in the code. We waited together silently as they opened up into the Alzheimer's ward. I signed in again at the nurse's station before proceeding to the activity room, and at this point Anne left me.

"Good luck," she said. "You'll need it." I wasn't sure if she was talking about the residents or my son, but she had flounced off down the hall before I could ask her.

Now I could hear screaming and yelling coming from the unit. Two of the residents were splayed up against the window looking out, making it difficult to get into the room. I banged on the door, hoping to catch an aide's attention. If there was a nurse around, she certainly wasn't in sight.

In fact, nobody was in sight. I pushed against the doors, and the two residents, Marge and Carl, backed off enough for me to get a foot in the door and force my way through.

And there they all were, either wandering around aimlessly or sitting in chairs; most of them looked blankly off into space. Gardner was in his usual spot. He liked to sit in the corner by the piano with his hand down his pants. He holds a Ph.D. in philosophy, but it's hard to believe sometimes. My personal favorite, Jerry, came up to greet me. He was holding a belt in his hand. "I don't know where this goes," he told me. I ignored him for the moment.

One of the activity assistants had already set up the tables at the far end of the room. They had been pushed together, and newspaper was spread out on top. A resident named Kate had started picking up some of the newspaper and was folding it into little squares. Golly, I thought to myself. It's going to be one of those days.

"Come on everybody," I yelled. "Let's sit down at the table."

I rolled a length of paper out along the table and began getting out brushes. Right then the doors burst open, and in rushed Kelly, the activity assistant. She looked flustered, but I needed her in the room with me to manage all these people, and I was relieved to see her. One by one she took them by the arm and led them over to the table where we would be painting. I began to sketch out a large Christmas tree with lots of presents at the bottom; it was large and simple. Patiently, Kelly placed a brush in one of their hands while I outlined the areas I wanted them to paint in.

I pour the paint into plastic drinking cups because it's easier to use and clean up afterward, but it can also be confusing for some people with dementia who might be thirsty. Today was no exception. "Carl is drinking the red paint," Kelly said. I turned around to see how much paint Carl had managed to swallow; he gave me a big grin, letting the paint run down both sides of his mouth. "He looks like a vampire," I said, and we both laughed.

"Who's going to report it to the nursing station?" I asked, "and who's going to clean him up?" I use non-toxic tempera paint because dementia patients sometimes drink anything they can get their hands on, and it's hard to watch eight residents all at the same time. "I'll fill out a report later," Kelly said, "and I'll clean him up, too. You just get the others started."

I turned back to the table. They were all seated now: Marge, the housewife; Jerry, who used to be a journalist; Kate, the diva; Granville, a CPA; Gardner, the college professor; George, the little retarded guy; and finally Mr. Bill, who swore up and down that he was a horse trainer at Pimlico Racetrack. No one knew if he had really trained horses or not because his paperwork always seemed to be missing. All of them must have had money at some time or another, or had a wealthy family member, because they were being housed at the most expensive facility in town. I found out that it cost over eight thousand dollars a month to keep them there, and all of them were private pays.

And now here they were, ready and waiting to paint a Christmas tree with me, just as if they could remember what Christmas was. So, I outlined each present carefully on one end, with lights and ornaments at the other end. I hoped they would paint inside the lines today, figuring I could always fill in any details that would be lost later. Kelly finally got Carl back to the table, and he was painting his name along the edge. His mouth had only faint pink marks now, but he was smiling.

"Hey, Kelly, you can give Carl high marks for active participation today. He's writing his name," I said. "Yeah, but what about Granville?" she asked. Granville was sitting up straight in his chair, but he had been poised with a brush full of green paint, not doing anything for over ten minutes, and I wasn't sure how to answer that.

"Granville, what are you doing?" I asked. He looked up at me and frowned.

"It's got to be done correctly," he answered.

"Just paint the tree, kiddo."

"They're making too many people," Granville said.

"Your mother wants one for her purse," Marge replied.

Strangely enough, working with them helped me forget my own troubles; it wasn't because I felt sorry for them, either. They were just damned funny.

"We are sitting here with all the children for lunch," Marge said.

They were all starting to babble and talk randomly, so I decided trying a different tactic to bring them back into the room with me and Kelly.

"Do you all want to hear the story about the time I painted with my mother?" I asked. The whole painting team looked up expectantly. They always loved to hear this story, which I repeated nearly every time I was there. I think that they enjoyed this particular story because they related to it on a very intimate basis; they knew me and now they knew my mother. I just kept reminding them that they knew.

"Your mother wants to hear it," Marge said.

"Well, did you know that my mom is in a nursing home?" I asked. They shook their heads up and down.

"Your mom is sick?" Jerry asked.

"Yes, dear, she can't walk or talk anymore."

"It's a damned shame," he said, then he put his head down in his hands, and he wouldn't look up. I wasn't sure if he was crying or not.

"Carl's drinking the paint again!" Kelly said.

"Well, at least it's the same color. You might not have to report it twice," I said. She got up and marched Carl into the bathroom once again. The group was still shifting around at the table. The Christmas tree had been quite forgotten.

Kate began to gather up all the newspaper. She had risen from her chair and was circling the table like an orbiting planet. "There's too many pieces," she said.

"Sit down, Kate, you want to hear the story," I commanded, and she sat down. I went over to Jerry then and pried his hands from his face.

"Jerry, dear, don't you want to hear the painting story?" I stood behind him and put both of my hands on either side of his shoulders. I wanted to make sure that he was emotionally stable.

"Oh, yes, yes. Is everyone in place for the meeting now?" he asked.

"Yes, we're all in place." I said. Now I could begin the story. When I felt that I had all of their attention, I began speaking.

"So, I drove my mom out into the field in my dad's Land Rover. The sun was bright, and the wind was blowing. It was a beautiful day. I got out the water bottle and the paint and the paper and the brushes, too."

"Do you have horses?" Mr. Bill asked.

"No, Bill, shut up," I said. "You're interrupting the story."

I started again. "I got my mom all ready to paint, and she looked at her watch and said, 'It's twelve o'clock.' And I said, 'So what? We're here to paint.' She told me that she always has lunch at twelve o'clock, and I told her that she's not having lunch today, she's painting instead. She starts to cry. You know I want my mom to be happy, so I pack everything back into the car."

"The table too?" Bill asked.

"Yes Bill, even the table. Then I drove out of the field and took her to get lunch. And after she had eaten lunch, I drove her back again so we could paint together."

"What about the table?" Bill asked.

"I told you, Bill, even the table. So, I got everything set

up again, and I got Mom positioned just right so that the sun wouldn't be in her eyes — and guess what she does?" I had all of their attention now; even Marge was leaning forward in her chair.

"She looked at her watch," I said.

"What time is it?" Kate asked.

"It was twelve o'clock again," I said. My mom always thinks it's twelve o'clock."

"Did she eat lunch?" Granville asked.

"No, this time she told me that she had to go to the bathroom." This brought laughter from the group because they could all relate to having to go to the bathroom. Jerry was laughing so much that he had dropped his paint brush and it fell into his lap. The brush had green paint on it, and now his crotch was green too. I hailed Kelly for the third time in an hour.

"Oh, Kelly, we've got another accident over here." She came around the table to where Jerry was sitting, pulling on her engagement ring. "When I get married to Norman, he says I don't have to work anymore." she said.

"Well, that's nice, dear. In the meantime, can you manage to get him cleaned up?" I asked.

I walked over to the table again and once more got paint brushes into everyone's hands. We started to paint again. Miraculously, they all stayed focused for the next 30 minutes or so, and we had what almost looked like a realistic version of a Christmas tree. Their families will be happy, I thought. All the families like to think that their relatives are busy doing things, as opposed to sitting in the hallways staring at the walls, Alzheimer's disease or not. I must admit, I can't blame them, either.

I looked at the clock and the hour was up. "And now it's time to clean up, gang," I said happily. Kelly came back again from the bathroom with evidence of green paint on her blouse. "I hate this job, but I need the money until I get married," she said. "Why do you keep coming back?"

"I guess I love what I do," I said.

"I think you're crazy," Kelly said.

"So everyone seems to be telling me today," I said. "Quite frankly, since you asked, I do enjoy working with these folks."

Kelly looked vague. "Yeah, I guess," she said, "but I'm getting out of here when I marry Norman." I decided to ignore her.

"Just don't forget to write in their charts about the paint." I said. I began to pack up my stuff and piled it back on the cart and turned to address the room at large. My dear students were all wandering off now; it was as if I hadn't even been there at all, save for the Christmas tree I had left behind.

"See you next week," I said, but nobody seemed to notice me leave.

I walked back out to my car, fortunately managing to avoid Anne on the way out of the building. She was in a meeting and looked up only briefly as I made my way down the hallway and through the doors. I opened the trunk of my rental car and began to load the art supplies. Just then my cell phone started to ring. The display indicated an out-of-state call. A chill went up my spine. I answered the phone, and it was my son Ben calling. I didn't even get a chance to say hello; he started to talk immediately.

"Mom, they won't let me go home. They've moved me to another place, and in 24 hours I won't have anywhere to go." He started to cry.

"Wait a minute, what's happened?"

I realized I was almost yelling. He stopped crying long enough to tell me that Debbie had called the social services in Collier County to report that he had tried to hurt the baby. A court order had been issued, stating that he couldn't go home again. Ben had nowhere else to go, was going to be released in 24 hours and would be out on the street by this time tomorrow. I thought about what Anne had said just an hour ago: "If it were my kid, I'd be on a plane by now."

"Where are you being held now?" I asked. He told me where he was and gave me the phone number. I scribbled it all down on the back of my hand with a permanent marker pen, the only thing I had in my pocket. Ben was sobbing again.

"Where am I going to go, what am I going to do?" he cried.

"I'm coming down to get you," I said.

"You don't even know where the place is," he lamented.

"Don't worry, I'll find you," I said, "but I have to hang up now. I've got to make some arrangements."

"I love you, Mom."

"I love you, too, son."

I climbed into the car and turned on the engine. I began making phone calls: first, the next nursing facility I was supposed to visit that afternoon, then all the places I had scheduled for the next day. I cancelled all my classes for a couple of days. Fortunately, everyone was very sympathetic. "Take the whole week off," one activity director told me. "Unfortunately, I can't. I need the money," I said. I drove the whole way home planning how I would get to Florida and wondering if I had enough left on my credit card for the plane fare.

One thing was certain: I was going to be cutting it close.

Chapter 7

December 7, 1999

It was very early in the morning, and I was driving my rental car down Falls Road toward the airport. In spite of not getting much sleep the night before, I felt more awake and alive than I could remember feeling in a long time. Maybe it was because I was finally able to do something about Ben, or maybe it was just plain fear. I was having difficulty telling the difference between fear and excitement. Either way, it seemed that not knowing the difference was definitely in my favor today. I looked down at my watch again. It was 5:00 a.m.

I did the math in my head: My plane left for Florida at 7:00 a.m., made one stop at Dulles airport, and arrived in Ft. Meyers at 2:18 p.m. I had to pick up a rental car and drive an hour to where my son was being held. That would take me up to 3:30 if I didn't get lost. The problem was that the last plane that day left at 4:53. How could I ever catch that last flight, and return a rental car?

After buying the plane tickets, there wasn't enough money left over to spend the night in Florida. I was broke, and my credit card had reached its limit. If I didn't get out on the last flight, Ben and I would be spending the night on the streets of Naples. Evelyn had given me $68 that she had set aside to buy Mickey new sneakers when she got up to see me off that morning.

"Here, take this money with you," she told me. "It's all the cash I've got on me, but you might need it for something. I think you need it more than we do."

"Thanks," I said. It has always been difficult for me to accept anything, and I felt especially humbled this morning. I was taking her kid's sneaker money, but I needed it. I crunched the bills into my back pocket and left by the back door. Evelyn followed me out into the gravel driveway, and I thanked her as best I could.

"I really do appreciate this, I'll pay you back as soon as I can," I said.

"Godspeed," was all she said, and then she went back into the old house.

The night before, after I'd made the flight reservations, I had called Debbie. I asked her if she could pick me up at the airport and explained about not having enough time to pick up Ben, drive back, and leave on the last flight. I also admitted that I didn't have enough money to spend the night.

"Can you help me?" I asked. Her reply was short and terse. "No," was what she said. I pressed on anyway.

"What about someone in your family?"

"We don't help people like you." Had she really said that?

I was stunned. A whole minute might have gone by before I could speak again.

"I'll remember that," I said.

"Go to hell," she said, and hung up.

And now my watch told me it was 5:10 a.m. The sky was just beginning to pale; pinky orange light was coming up in the east, dark blue clouds drifted along closer to the horizon. I could just make out the outline of the city. *"I'm coming, Bubba. I'm coming to get you"* was the only thing running through my head.

It took exactly 43 minutes to drive to the airport, a fact I knew from checking my watch every minute or so. As I swung the car into the long-term parking lot I could see a transport bus a couple of rows away. A short line of people waited to board. I was traveling light. I had two empty suitcases and a book titled *Living with a Schizophrenic*. The suitcases would be used to pack whatever clothes Ben had managed to salvage from his belongings. My money, credit card, and driver's license were all crammed in the back pocket of my jeans.

I jumped out of the car, grabbed the two suitcases, and slammed the door, keeping my eye on the bus. It hadn't left yet, and I ran toward it. "Wait for me, wait!" I yelled. I ran desperately toward the open door and was able to climb the few steps into the relative warmth inside. Two rows of people, already seated, looked up at me as the bus took off. There was standing room only, and I grabbed a hand grip that hung from a vertical bar. *"I'm coming, Bubba, I'm coming."*

I didn't have any bags to check, so I got a boarding pass outside the terminal, walked through the automatic doors, and went directly over to the screen showing departures and arrivals. My flight was scheduled to leave at 6:58 a.m., giving me almost an hour to wait.

By the time I found the gate and sank into a chair, the gravity of my situation overwhelmed me. The excitement of leaving and driving to the airport had now transformed into fear. It was hard to breathe. The possibility of having to spend the night without funds in a strange city took my breath away. Now it was 6:15. Who would reassure me that I was doing the right thing? And Gertrude came to mind. It was a silly notion, actually. I had just met the old woman. She didn't even know me or anything about my situation. What was I going to say? "Hi, this is your art teacher, and I need some advice"? She'd think I was out of my mind, but I remembered what she had told me the day before.

"I pray for people," she had said. "I pray for people and they get better."

I knew that she had her own phone, and I knew her number. I could see two pay phones from where I sat, and nobody was using either one. I had nothing to lose, nothing in the world. I had already sold everything worth anything, was down to a rental car and $68 in my pocket. What the heck — if I woke her up, she was a good Catholic and might forgive me, or she might forget my phone call within ten minutes. She had dementia. Either way, I still had nothing to lose.

I got up slowly and walked to the phone. I dropped a quarter into the slot and dialed Gertrude's number. It rang six times before she answered. I know because I was holding my breath and counting the rings.

"Hello?"

"Gertrude, this is your art teacher." I was breathless again.

"It's who?"

"It's your art teacher."

"What time is it?" she asked. "I'm still in bed. Did I oversleep again?"

"No, no, it's very early, Gertrude. I am calling to ask you a favor."

"Are you coming today, dear?" She sounded so sweet, just like a wonderful fairy godmother. I could imagine her in the little bed with pink blankets covering her and the black plastic rosary on top of the covers.

"No, actually I'm at the airport, Gertrude. I'm going to Florida today to pick up my son, Ben. He's in trouble and I need to help him."

"Oh my," Gertrude said. I could hear her shifting around now. She was probably arranging her granny cap and taking a drink of water from the glass she kept beside her bed. Maybe she was getting out the rosary beads.

"I have a favor to ask of you," I said. She was still shifting around, and I wasn't sure if she had heard me. "Did you hear me Gertrude?"

"Yes, dear, what is it?" she asked.

I took another gulp of air. I had very little money and not enough time to get my son and come home today. What I needed was direct intervention of the supernatural kind. Gertrude was my best shot — in fact, she was my only shot.

"I need you to pray for me and Ben, that we'll get home tonight," I stammered.

"Why, of course I will, dear. Why, I'll start right now, and you have a nice day," she said. Then she hung up before I could explain anything further. Oh good God, what if she doesn't remember? I hung up the phone just in time to hear my flight called. I would be boarding soon, flying off into a strange void, not knowing whether I could even get back — and I was going anyway.

Maybe Kelly was right after all, maybe I *was* crazy. I had just called an 88-year-old woman with dementia. Worse still, maybe there was no God after all, at least not one who heard petty troubles. But there wasn't time to mull this over or even cry. My plane was boarding and the die was cast; I was going to Florida, come hell or high water.

The little plane held only 16 people, and the pilot served as the flight attendant as well. "There won't be complimentary services," he told us. "The plane won't be in the air long enough." I looked around. The plane was filled with businessmen going to Washington, D.C. Most had on dark suits and carried briefcases. The only other woman sat down next to me.

She was at least as old as Gertrude and carried a large brown paper bag that held her shawl and her lunch. I found this out because she kept up a steady monologue during the entire flight. She also told me that she was scared to fly, and every time the plane took a dip or a turn she would gasp and grab my hand.

"Pray with me," she demanded, "so we won't be killed!"

The plane touched down at 8:15a.m. and rolled to a complete stop. It was a puddle-jumper and couldn't dock at the terminal; instead, a crew of two men rolled a metal staircase out onto the airfield and right up to the door of our plane. My old lady companion began to whine and wring her hands.

"I'm afraid of heights," she cried. "What if I fall and break my leg on those awful stairs?"

"Don't worry, I'll help you," I said. So together we made it down the metal stairs. I held her arm as we crossed the airfield and went into the Dulles terminal. She was met almost immediately by a scraggly group of apparent family members who greeted her as if she were the queen of England. For a brief moment I was jealous of her. She had a family, and I was by myself.

I ambled along the concourse and found another information panel. My flight was still scheduled to leave on time for Ft. Meyers. It would be leaving Dulles at 11:45a.m.. I had about three hours to wait for the plane. I thought how ironic it all was. Here was a gap of three hours, and all I was asking for was 20 minutes. I had done the math again, and I was positive that if the flight took off 20 minutes early I would have just enough time to find Ben and get home...today.

My stomach was rumbling, but I decided not to spend any of the sneaker money, just in case I would need to get something for Ben later on. Instead I sat down in front of a television and opened my book on schizophrenia. I was interested in the weather forecast for Ft. Meyers and Naples, hoping for sunshine. I didn't think I would be able to take it if we had to walk around the city all night long in the rain. It hadn't occurred to me to bring an umbrella.

I opened the book and started to read, intermittently watching the weather channel. I don't know how long I sat there. I must have looked odd or perhaps interesting at the very least, because after a while a man came up and asked if I was OK. He was dressed in a tan uniform with a United Air patch on his sleeve. A plastic name badge hung around his neck; he looked official.

"I've never seen anyone read and watch TV at the same time before," he said. I looked up from my book.

"Are you talking to me?" I asked.

"Yes, Miss," he said, and then he added, "Are you all right?" He looked inquisitive and concerned. My first impulse was to say I was fine and to move along. I closed the book, started to gather my empty bags, and stood up. We were face to face now; he hadn't moved an inch. "I'm fine," I said, and then I sat back down and opened the book again to indicate that our conversation was over.

"Are you a therapist or something?" he asked.

"Why would you think that?" I asked in turn. He pointed at the book in my lap.

"In my opinion schizophrenia isn't necessarily a topic anyone would read unless they were a therapist or something like that," he said. I thought, *what's it going to take to get rid of this guy?* I can't remember why I decided to tell him the reason I was going to Florida. Maybe it was only because he was somebody to talk to, and I was afraid and alone; at any rate, I spilled the beans. I told him all about Ben and why I had to make a heroic effort and bring him back to Baltimore.

"Gee," he said, "I bet you could really use a cigarette."

"Yeah, right, but we're in Dulles airport, and there's a no-smoking rule," I said.

He patted his badge knowingly. "True for most, but I work for United Airlines, and we've got an area where the pilots and flight attendants can smoke," he said. "Interested?" I looked down at my watch to check the time. There was still over an hour before my flight left.

"Of course," I told him.

"Then follow me."

I normally don't take up with strangers, but I had already embarked on a wild enough adventure to rescue Ben, so what did I have to lose? I followed him. He led me back to the gate area, and we walked down one of the corridors that lead out to the planes. Instead of getting on a plane, though, we went down another metal staircase that led out to the field. Then we walked around the side of the building where there was an area fenced in with chicken wire. It formed a kind of cage. There were several pilots and flight attendants standing around an old oil drum smoking cigarettes.

The scene had an end-of-the-world quality about it, because the whole enclosure was rusted and dilapidated. As I got closer, I could see that the oil drum had been filled with dirt to serve as a gigantic ashtray. In direct contrast to the wire contraption, the pilots looked brand-new and crisp in their navy blue uniforms. My companion said hello to a couple of them and then threw his arm around me in a familial gesture indicating that I had clearance. He reached into his pocket, pulled out a pack of Kool Filter Kings and handed me one. I only smoke occasionally, but I gratefully took it anyway.

"This is wonderful," I said. I was beginning to think that Gertrude must be praying for me by now. After all, it looked as if I had been granted a smoke break by the Almighty.

My new friend finished his cigarette and threw it into the oil drum. "Good luck with your son," he said. "I've got to get back to work, but if there's anything else I can do, let me know."

I laughed at this. My predicament was staggering to me. I continued to giggle from the absurdity of his offer. "What's so funny?" he asked. He looked perplexed now.

"Listen, what I need you can't give me," I replied.

"And that is?"

"I need to land in Ft. Meyers 20 minutes before schedule to have enough time to pick up my son, then get back to the airport and come home, all in the same day. I'm sort of flying on a wing and a prayer," I finished.

He smiled. "Then today is your lucky day." He pulled a radio phone from a belt that was fastened about his waist and began talking to someone. I was still baffled.

"What do you mean?" I asked. He put the phone back into his belt and began talking, but I couldn't hear anything he was saying. It was a windy day, and a big jet was taxiing up the field toward us. The roar of the engines drowned out everything he was saying. I stepped closer. "I can't hear you!" I yelled.

He didn't answer me, just started to make arm motions that indicated I should follow him. He seemed to be heading back to the terminal, so I followed behind. It was 11:05 a.m.

I followed him through a side door and realized that we had arrived at my gate. The waiting area was jammed with people, and the sign was lit up in red for Ft. Meyers. Many people were already standing in a line waiting to get boarding passes. He stopped there and pulled out his phone, but, again, I couldn't hear what he was saying. The jet engines from out on the field were still roaring in my ears. He finally got off the phone and turned back to me. "Your flight is leaving early — you better get going," he said. I was incredulous. I heard what he said, but I felt as if my feet were cemented to the floor. I couldn't move.

"What do you mean? How can it leave early?" I asked. His smile was broad this time; I could see all of his teeth. He seemed happy to be informing me of this new turn of events. *Oh, my God, I have been following a crazy person around the airport.* I thought I was going to have to start screaming for a security guard to save me, but he went on to explain.

"I'm in charge of scheduling outbound flights for United Air," he said. "And you will be landing in Ft. Meyers at 2:00 p.m."

"What about the other passengers?" I asked. He held up the radio phone for me to see.

"I've been in communication with the flight attendant over there." He waved his hand toward the desk where the attendant was handing out boarding passes. "Everyone's either here or accounted for, and if I were you, I'd get in line, United Air flight 547 will be leaving soon."

"I don't know what to say. How can I thank you?" I asked.

"Just take care of your son and God bless you both," he said. We shook hands, and I turned to get in line with the other passengers. Funny thing was, it didn't even occur to me until I was in the air that a miracle had just happened. My spirits were now soaring along with the plane. For the first time in over a week I knew that Ben was going to be OK.

Chapter 8

December 8, 1999

Ben had left most of his things in Florida, and the next day he borrowed one of my big, heavy sweaters and went outside. The sun was out, but there was a chill in the air. The grass on the front lawn was a brilliant green. I looked out the window from the kitchen to check on him.. It made me nervous to see him out on the lawn. Now that we had made it back to Baltimore, I didn't want to lose him.

He had been emotional on the way home and seemed disoriented. I hadn't been prepared for that. Fortunately though, we'd been served a hearty snack on the flight home, and I'd used some of Mickey's sneaker money to buy us both a beer. That had calmed me, and Ben fell asleep.

Now it was Wednesday morning, and Evelyn had driven Mickey to school, so Ben and I had the kitchen to ourselves for the time being. My plan was to take him to the emergency room at the hospital since he was no longer under the care of a doctor. It was the only way to have him evaluated. Under the circumstances, I didn't know whether he was going to need a psychiatrist or a neurosurgeon.

There wasn't much in the refrigerator to fix for breakfast. There never seemed to be anything to eat, in spite of the fact that I went grocery shopping all the time. It was one of those roommate details that Evelyn and I hadn't worked out yet, and I was beginning to resent it, especially this morning. I decided not to speak with her about it yet, though. Sixty of Mickey's sneaker dollars still remained in my possession.

I made toast and coffee, and we got ourselves together in no time at all. Before I knew it, we were in the car, back on the same route I had taken the day before, driving south into Baltimore. I reasoned that if we got there early enough, we wouldn't have to wait so long. But I was wrong. A very overweight nurse brought us into a small room to do what she called an "intake." We squeezed in with her, but her immense size made it feel more like a broom closet than a room. Her main concern seemed to be insurance: whether Ben had any, what was the company's name, address, and so forth. It wasn't until these criteria had been established that she began to take his pulse, blood pressure, and the like. After that, the interview process got a little sticky. She asked Ben the questions, and I answered them.

"Exactly why are you here today?" she asked.

"He tried to commit suicide," I replied. She seemed perfectly calm about this, never looking up, writing it down in a little box on her chart.

"When and where did this suicide attempt take place?" she asked.

"Right before Thanksgiving, in . . ."

She cut me off in mid-sentence. "I believe that Ben is an adult and can answer the questions himself," she said. "Why don't you take a seat in the waiting room please?"

"I am staying right here," I said, and then, as an afterthought added, "you'll need me to fill in his medical history." At this Ben began to nod his head in agreement.

"I'm a little fuzzy," he said. I had to agree with that. Actually, we both looked a little worse for wear. He had a day's growth of beard, and my striped sweater looked completely out of place over the gray sweat pants he had pulled on earlier that morning. As for me, I had yanked my hair back into a ponytail and was wearing my old leather jacket with yesterday's jeans. My hiking boots were muddy, and one of Ben's sneakers had a hole in the toe. We must have looked crumpled at best.

The nurse looked at both of us then and probably summed up the situation for herself, because all she said was, "Suit yourselves." In the end, it took us over an hour to recount the circumstances that had led us to the emergency room that morning. The nurse had softened considerably. She even let me answer some of the questions. Finally she led us to another room and told Ben to go in, take off his clothes, and put on a hospital gown. Then she gave me my instructions.

"There's a cafeteria on the fifth floor. Why don't you go get a cup of coffee?" she suggested. "We'll need to take a CAT scan before we can determine anything, and it will be a while." She wasn't wrong about that. Six hours later, Ben and I were still waiting. It was two o'clock in the afternoon, and I had drunk at least 10 cups of coffee. I called Elliott and asked him to come over to the hospital and bring some sandwiches. He taught art at a private school but didn't have regular hours and usually had ample time in the afternoon. I wanted him to relieve me and hang out with Ben for a while. Even though I am used to being in hospitals, it's a vastly different experience when it's your own kid.

Elliott showed up 45 minutes later carrying a bag full of oranges and some candy bars. "What the hell is this crap, Elliott?" I asked. "Did you rob an old lady on the way here? I was thinking more along the lines of a submarine sandwich and some magazines." My nerves were fried, and I was getting testy.

"Hey, take a break and get off my ass," Elliott said. "I'm doing the best I can!"

He pushed me out of the room and into the hall. Suddenly we were standing in the middle of chaos. Bells were ringing, and doctors and nurses were rushing from one patient to another. The place was packed with humanity and noise. Many of the patients were separated only by sheer white curtains that hung from tracks in the ceiling. "You better get your shit together," he said. "Ben needs you." He was right, of course, but I was tired and scared. We had been in the emergency room for a long time, and I had run completely out of patience.

"I can't just stand around anymore!" I told him. "What am I going to do now?"

"Listen, take a walk or something. I'll stay here with Ben," he suggested.

I looked up and down the hall, hoping to catch the doctor who had seen Ben earlier. We were still waiting to hear about the results of the CAT scan. Not knowing anything has always been worse for me than hearing bad news. "I'm going to wander around and see what I can find out from the doctor," I told Elliott. "I'll be back soon."

"Take your time," he said. "Ben is sleeping anyway, but I'll be here if he wakes up."

I walked down the hall and turned left where earlier I had seen several doctors in white lab coats looking at x-rays on backlit screens. That area was empty now, so I just kept following signs that read "Special Imaging."

No one paid any attention to me, so I kept going, hoping to find somebody who could tell me something — anything. I took another left and found myself in a brightly lit corridor where two men, both in white lab coats, were standing and talking together. One man had a gray beard. Seen in profile, he looked vaguely familiar, yet I couldn't place where I had seen him before. I was trying to remember when they both turned toward me. Now I could see his face clearly. He was smiling; then I remembered.

"Richard! Is that you?" We were both taken by surprise.

"What are you doing here?" he asked. He walked toward me, and we shook hands. "I thought you were a college professor or something," I said. At this, he threw his head back and laughed. His colleague must have thought this was funny, because he started laughing, too. Richard dismissed him.

"I'll talk with you about that case later," he said. His colleague turned and left, but he was still chuckling. We were alone in the corridor now.

"So what are you doing here?" he asked.

"My son had a CAT scan earlier today. We've been waiting for hours, and I thought I'd try to find a doctor who could tell me what's going on," I said.

I started to cry then. I didn't want to cry, but there I was, crying in the corridor. Little hiccups were coming out of my throat. I felt stupid and ashamed. I barely knew this man. Richard put his arm around my shoulders.

"Don't fret, I'm a radiologist," he said. "Let's go find those films and see what's going on."

"I thought you were a history professor," I said.

He grinned. "Whatever made you think that?" he asked.

"I think it's the beard," I said.

And so he led me back down the hall, to the wall of illuminated x-rays. Beneath that wall was a long bench, and on the bench was a tall stack of oversized envelopes. Richard shuffled through them and, after a few minutes, found what he was looking for. He pulled a large negative out of the envelope he had selected and put it up on the lighted screen. To me, it looked like a lot of black, gray, and white blobs. I watched his profile as he surveyed the screen. He was a handsome man, but the gray beard made him look older than he probably was.

"There are five areas in question here," he said. "The little bleeds could very well be artifacts from an earlier time. Does your son have a history of seizure activity?"

"Yes, we were here about a year ago, but nothing was conclusive. I wanted him to get more tests, but he moved out of state before that could happen."

"Why?"

"It's a very long story, Richard. I'll tell you about it some other time, but the point is what should I do today?"

"I'm going to call up the film library and see what we have on file. I want to compare films and see what, if anything, has changed. Then we'll determine what to do." he said. Now I interrupted him.

"He tried to kill himself," I said.

Richard frowned. "I think you'll need to tell me more," he said.

I never got the chance to tell him the story, though. Before I could relay another thing, he was paged. I understood all too well. He was a doctor and probably had a hundred patients to see that day, yet he had gone out of his way to help me. He seemed to be one of those rare individuals who are kind to others, no matter where you meet them or what the circumstances are. On the first occasion I had met him – and even now — I felt better just being around him.

I turned to go, and he touched my arm. "I'll look at those films as soon as I can," he said. "Why don't you go get yourself a cup of coffee in the meantime?"

"It seems as if everyone's been telling me to drink coffee all day," I said. Then I thanked him again for taking the time to talk with me.

"It's my pleasure," he said, before leaving me alone in the hallway.

I looked at all the black and white blobs on the film in front of me. It was a mystery to me what it meant. Finally I went back to find Elliott and Ben. I'd been missing long enough. As I walked back to Ben's room, I thought to myself, *He's a great guy, but after today I'll probably never see him again.*

Much later the emergency room doctor gave us the report. There would be no need to operate, but he and the other doctors recommended that Ben spend some time in the psychiatric hospital for evaluation and stabilization. It was 8:00 p.m., and we had spent the last 11 hours in the emergency room. Elliott had left earlier to teach his night class, so Ben and I received the news together.

"Can you come with me, Mom?" he asked. "I don't want to go to another hospital by myself."

"I can't go with you this time, son," I said, "but I promise to see you tomorrow after work. They're going to transport you in the ambulance. It's some kind of hospital regulation, and I can't come along." He looked down at his hands and began to cry.

"I miss my son," he said.
"I know dear, so do I."

Thursday, December 9, 1999

Once Ben was institutionalized and safe for the immediate time, I was able to get back to work — a relief for me. I reasoned that if I could get back into my normal routine, life would get easier and the crisis over, at least soon. This was my general attitude as I started the week's business again. My first client on Thursday morning that week was Gertrude, I was eager to see her, and I wanted to talk to her about what had happened. And I needed to thank her for the help that had come my way. I drove down her street with the fish ponds in the middle. The fountains had been turned off for the winter. Mallard ducks were swimming, and a couple of workers were cleaning dead leaves out of the ponds. Everything seemed to be in order there, and I enjoyed the view. I wondered what it would be like to live on a street where everything seemed perfect. I drove around to the alley behind the Professor's house and parked my car. They had given me a key to the house. The Mrs. had told me earlier that she would be in meetings all week long and to let myself in. I had another duty: to make Gertrude lunch before I left. The nurse practitioner had given explicit instructions about what lunch should consist of: a small bunch of grapes, three slices of American cheese, a bran muffin, a glass of milk, and a cup of hot tea. There was a list waiting for me on the kitchen counter on top of a brown serving tray. I read the list while I looked around the kitchen. The Mrs. collected roosters; they were everywhere.

The dog met me halfway up the stairs to Gertrude's room; otherwise, the house was empty. I knocked on the door to her room, got no response, and knocked again. I waited with the dog in the hall with no answer. Finally, I pushed the door open and went in. The room was dark as a bat's cave. I couldn't see a thing until I found the light switch and turned it on. Now I could see that Gertrude was still in bed — and it was almost noon.

A breakfast tray on the card table held a bowl of cereal, a large glass of milk, half a banana, and a handful of assorted medications. Little pink capsules, long white pills, a tiny round caplet that had been broken in half, and some clear gel caps were lying in a cup on the side of the tray. While I was checking out her tray, the dog had managed to climb up onto Gertrude's bed and was licking her face. She moaned and turned over on her side, away from me. She had rolled toward the wall, exposing lumpy bed linens and a stack of *Good Housekeeping* magazines underneath a pile of blankets near the foot of her bed.

One thing was certain: She didn't look like anyone who could elicit the attention of God. I didn't know much about miracles then; the only link I had to God or religion had been through my paternal grandmother, Fanny. She used to tell me that God worked in mysterious ways. From the look of things, this seemed as true today as it had been when my grandmother had pronounced it.

I cleared my throat and walked over to where Gertrude was lying. I stood directly over her. The dog had jumped down to the floor now and rolled onto his back, begging to have his stomach rubbed. I pushed him aside with my foot; he squealed and barked. The commotion woke Gertrude, and she sat straight up. A plastic rosary fell to the floor. Suddenly we were face to face. She was surprised to see me.

"What are you doing here?" she asked, rubbing her eyes.

"It's my day," I said. She looked baffled at first, and then I could see realization dawning on her face.

"Ah, yes, you're my art teacher. Well, missy, I'm not painting now. You'll have to come back later today."

I felt a jab of anger. Who did she think she was, anyway? She just couldn't order me around. I had a schedule to keep. Other patients were waiting to see me, too. I told her this.

"Well, change your schedule!" she said. Her jaw jutted out in disgust as she rose from the bed. "Don't just stand there, get my walker!" At that point it seemed easier to get her the walker rather than argue. I complied. She got behind the walker and proceeded to walk to the door of her room. Now I was confused.

"Where are you going?" I asked.

"I'm going to use the facilities. Now get out of my way!" she cried. And with that, she pushed herself out the door and toward the bathroom down the hall. I was left with the dog, who had come over to sit by my side. He seemed to be grinning up at me.

While I waited for Gertrude, I surveyed her room. Most of the dresser drawers were pulled out, revealing an incredible variety of materials, clothes, books, and boxes inside. I edged my way over to get a better view of the contents, hoping that she would take awhile in the bathroom and not catch me looking through her stuff. In one drawer, a pile of stockings had been tied into knots, and beneath that was an old photo album. The cracked red leather cover looked as if it had been opened thousands of times.

Gingerly, I pulled the red album out from under the stockings and opened it.

Inside, the pages were crumbling. The few faded photos were all black and white. A pretty little girl with dark hair, squinting, was wearing a white dress. On the back of the photograph: "1947, Jane's first communion." I guessed from the date that the little girl must be Gertrude's daughter. I shuffled through the album, looking for other pictures from her past, but could only find two others that were of any interest. One was a wallet-sized wedding photo, and one of a much-younger Gertrude with a fancy hat, standing in front of a white porch. It might have been Easter, judging from the little flowers coming up in the grass. Gertrude was holding a purse, wore white gloves, and gave the impression that she was going somewhere special, maybe church.

These images supported my idea that she was religious.

Suddenly I was startled back into the present. I could hear Gertrude coming back down the hall. Her walker scraped as she pushed it over the carpet. I shoved the red album back under the stockings and made certain that it all looked as I had found it. I stepped back from the dresser just in time. She slammed her way into the doorway, hitting the door frame with the walker. She was stuck.

"Help me, for God's sake! Don't just stand there," she yelled. Quickly I moved over to the door and opened it wider so she could enter her room. I felt guilty about snooping through her stuff. She made her way directly over to the card table with the breakfast tray. She sat down in her wheelchair and started to pour milk on the cereal. She acted as if I weren't even there! I sat down in a folding chair by the table. I didn't know what else to do.

Gertrude reached over and patted my hand. "Don't worry, child, I really don't care if we paint at all." Then she cut the banana into little pieces. "I haven't had my breakfast yet," she told me, as if that would explain everything.

I glanced over at the clock; it said 1:09 p.m. It was a large digital clock with bright red numbers that anyone could see clearly from the other end of a football field. I had another 20 minutes until I could leave, and we hadn't painted a thing.

"Let's paint a basket," I said. Where had that come from?

"You want to do magic?" she asked.

I rolled my eyes at this remark before I realized that she wasn't hearing me. I tried again.

"Let's paint instead!" I was almost yelling now.

"You want me to go to bed?" she asked.

"Never mind, just eat your cereal," I said.

"Thank you, dear. I'll just finish my breakfast," she said. Gertrude sat back in her chair and smiled graciously at me. She looked angelic, not like the old lady who had just acted as if I weren't even there.

She continued to eat her cereal as I had suggested, and we didn't paint anything that day. I left early, not caring if she liked it or not. Gertrude didn't pay any attention to me until I was almost out the door. I had my hand on the doorknob, making my exit, when she spoke again.

"Oh, missy," she smiled, sweetly now, "I have a bit of advice to impart."

I turned around to better hear what Gertrude was going to tell me. She held up her spoon filled with bran cereal and spilling over with milk. She didn't seem to notice the milk dribbling on her bathrobe. Instead, her eyes were fixed on me. The dog sat beside her, and I will swear until this day that he was still grinning at me. I waited by the door, my anticipation heightened by the long pause.

"Live and learn," she said.

I closed her door behind me and quietly descended the stairs, sighing relief.

My next stop was the hospital. I took my time getting there. The traffic was relatively calm at this time of day, and I didn't feel I had to rush. I had all the time in the world. I had left Gertrude's house sooner than expected, arriving five minutes early by the time I pulled into the hospital's parking lot. For some reason or another, five minutes seemed like a lot of time to spend with myself. I sat in the car, letting the engine run, feeling the hot air coming through the vents on the floor. It felt warm, wonderful, and good. But I was morose.

I looked up to the second floor, toward Park Unit. Already, there were several of my patients looking out the front windows and waving at me. I was tired, but I couldn't tell them that, now could I? No. I felt that my life had suddenly taken a radical turn for the worse in every possible way. I felt miserable and alone in the world. The problem was, I couldn't share any of my feelings. For one thing, I needed to be strong for Ben. I didn't trust anyone else, for another. It seemed it had always been this way and would always be this way; for ever and ever, amen. I always ended up having to go though crises by myself. I started thinking how unfair life had been to me.

Already the sun was getting lower in the sky, and there was a chill in the air. On the western side of the street was a pale pink-orange glow near the horizon. In front of the hospital, several men were hanging tiny white lights in the trees. Turned on, the strings of lights looked surrealistic; some of them were still spread out all over the lawn. Small, elfin men in brown uniforms bent over the lights. I looked at my watch. My five minutes were up. I got out of the warm car and walked into the hospital.

Inside the front lobby, the entire activity staff was busy pulling green pine boughs from boxes scattered all over the floor. "I'll Be Home for Christmas" was playing on a portable radio, and the atmosphere was ... jolly. The activities cart was parked off to one side of the lobby, filled with large containers of paint. Alex saw me first and jumped up from where he had been unraveling a bundle of Christmas tree lights.

"They're all ready for you upstairs," he said. "I'll be along in a minute."

"See you up there," I said.

I pushed the cart in front of me and got into the elevator to go up to Park Unit. There seemed to be tinsel everywhere, but it only made me feel more depressed. Once I got off on the second floor, though, I could hear children singing all the way down the hall, their voices high pitched, bright, slightly off-key. I pushed the cart, slowing, down the hall, hoping they would finish soon, and waited behind the tables that had already been set up.

The children's teacher must have known that I was next on the activity agenda, because, as soon as she saw me come into the room, she stopped playing and began to gather them into a tight little group. The children looked up at me expectantly. I felt as if I should say something nice to them since none of the activity personnel was around to wrap things up.

"Good show," I said, thinking to myself how pitiful they really were.

The teacher looked me straight in the eye, almost as if she already knew I could care less, and folded her hands in front of her. "Thank you. We've been practicing for weeks," she said. Now I felt worse. I had managed to insult little children and their teacher with my attitude alone. I was mulling this over when suddenly someone's hand came down on my shoulder. Startled, I turned around.

"What's up, girl?" It was a cheerful voice. It was Alex. He

was wearing a red Santa hat and smiling broadly. Before I could say anything, he had walked past me and started to move people into their places around the tables. There were 20 people or so left over from the singing assembly, and Alex was whistling happily as he worked. He turned away from the patients and spoke to me.

"Hey, Sister Marie was wondering if they could paint a Christmas mural today," Alex said.

"What kind of Christmas mural?" I asked. "The manger scene, a Christmas tree, or do we have to do something politically correct?"

"What's your problem? This is a Catholic hospital, remember?" he replied.

"Whatever you want — I'm your trusted servant," I said and bowed.

Then I heard something I couldn't quite make out. I turned my attention to the people parked around the tables in their wheelchairs. Was someone talking to me? Betty was the closest, and she was looking over at Mary across the table. "You're a real asshole," she said again.

"Screw you too," Mary said back.

I didn't feel like breaking up an argument, so I walked behind Betty and put both my hands on her shoulders. "What's going on?" I asked.

"Wassa matter wi you?" she asked, looking up at me.

"My oldest kid is sick," I told her.

"My husband just up and died two year ago. I kinda hate this time o' year too," she said. Then she reached out and put her one good hand on my arm.

"The Lord giveth and the Lord taketh away," she said.

The poignancy of her words caught me off guard. She had touched upon my deeper fear: My son could die. Nervously, I started to laugh, and then she began to laugh too. "You've really cheered me up this time," I said.

"What's so funny? Are you laughing at me?" Mary asked. Betty leaned forward in her chair. She pulled her stick out from under the blanket on her lap and shook it at Mary.

"I'm gonna knock yo silly head off," she threatened. "Her chile is sick."

"That's enough out of both of you," I told them. "Let's not fight. I'm here to paint the manger scene. Are you going to help with this project or continue to argue?"

"Let's paint!" Betty yelled.

"My head hurts," Mary cried.

"Just shut up and paint, Mary. I'm really not in the mood today for your whining, OK?" She looked down at her hands.

"I don't want to paint today," she said.

"Fine," I said. "That's just fine."

My next stop was the psychiatric hospital where Ben was staying. The hospital was on my way home, and I was making my first attempt to visit him. It had been 24 hours since I had left him in the emergency room. It was already nightfall, and the sky was now dark blue. I could see the lighted windows in the hospital and wondered which room was his. I knew Ben was in one of the special care units, but I didn't know where to go.

I pulled into a parking lot closest to the road and looked around again. One sign said Administration and another pointed to Adult Residential. I decided to go in on the residential side. A young girl working the front desk gave me directions. She was very upbeat and happy; I resented her immediately. She gave me a printed sheet of general information and pointed me toward a long hallway.

"Go down there and turn left," she said.

I managed to get lost right away by walking down a series of long halls that led me far into the back of the building. It was like a maze, with halls going around corners and then bending back again. I was fairly certain that I had passed the same cork board twice. An old woman stood near a short flight of stairs, leaning on a broom and watching me.

"You look like you're lost." she said. "Whatcha looking for?"

"Park Unit," I told her.

"There ain't no Park Unit," she replied.

"Gee, I'm sorry. It's been a long day. I'm looking for the special care unit on the second floor." I said.

The old lady smiled knowingly and pointed at some stairs. "Go to the top, turn left, and you'll walk right into it."

I thanked her and climbed the stairs. I felt about 90 years old. I was very tired. When I got to the top of the stairs, I turned left and nearly crashed into a door with frosted glass in the top panel. There was a doorbell off to one side. A hand-written message in red ink read "Ring for entry." Behind the frosted glass I could make out shadowy forms. I rang the bell. Almost immediately, several dark forms approached the door from the other side. Then the door opened inward. I heard a male voice say "Get back," and then, "Just a minute." I didn't know if the voice was talking to me or the forms on the other side of the door, so I waited to see what would happen next.

The door opened wider, and someone said "Well, come on, don't just stand there." I pushed in and found myself in another long corridor. This one was filled with people, some wearing white uniforms. Two uniformed men were herding several people back down this hallway. I, on the other hand was commanded to a stop by a woman I took to be the charge nurse.

"Give me your purse and your coat," she commanded. Grudgingly I handed my belongings over to a young man who had just emerged from a nearby room. I assumed this was an office, although it looked very unusual; it had many shelves stacked with cigarettes, hair spray and perfume, stockings and toilet paper.

"What patient are you here to visit?" the nurse asked. She was holding a clipboard, anticipating my answer. Her pen was poised, but I was having a hard time staying focused. I had become distracted by the young man, who had started to rummage through my things. He had taken a cigarette lighter out of my purse and was placing it into a plastic bag.

"What is going on here?" I asked the nurse.

She looked at me over the top of her glasses and sighed. Then she went on to explain that they searched everyone's belongings for hair spray, cigarettes, matches, knives, fingernail files, and the like. Apparently all of these things were potential hazards for people who had recently been trying to kill themselves. "This ward is *restricted*," she said to illustrate her point. Suddenly I understood the contents of the shelves in the office.

"What is the patient's name?" She asked.

"Ben, his name is Ben," I said.

She looked down at her clipboard again and then back at me. "I'll be sure to inform him that you came to visit, but you can't see him yet. He's still in isolation," she said.

"But I'm his mother," I told her.

"I'm sorry, but he can't have any visitors yet. Please call first next time," she said.

Suddenly we were interrupted by a ruckus down the hall. A young girl was trying to hit one of the men in white. The nurse gave me her card, ignoring the commotion. "Here is the number for the hospital and the extension for this unit. It's time for you to leave now," she said.

The young man came out of the strange little office carrying my purse and coat. These he handed back over to me. I was gently shoved back out the main door with the frosted panel. It closed behind me with a great thud. I didn't know what else I could do, so I just went back down the stairs.

I was met again by the old lady with the broom. "Merry Christmas," she said.

Chapter 9

December 27, 1999

Somehow I managed to get through the holidays, but it was rough going. I spent most of my time jockeying myself between work, visiting Ben, and driving to and from Baltimore and my place in the country. I spent Christmas day with Ben in the psych unit, but there wasn't much said between us, and I had so little money that I ended up sharing dinner off his tray instead of getting something to eat on the way home.

Ben and the other patients had fashioned ornaments from pipe cleaners and construction paper. These makeshift pieces adorned a large, tipsy tree that had been set up in one corner of the common room. Colored lights had been thrown in a random fashion over the top of the tree. To me it seemed a half-hearted attempt, and the overall effect was depressing

My dementia patients, on the other hand, had made beautiful ornaments from wallpaper and glitter. We had created handmade soaps, decorated candles, and painted large murals of holiday trees. We made entire Christmas villages out of cardboard boxes. I had had two conversations with the nurses on Ben's unit about the lack of activity programs for him and the other patients.

"What do they do during the day?" I asked.

"We engage with patients in group sessions several times a day," the nurse explained.

"What exactly does this accomplish?" I asked. The nurse looked indignant and folded her arms across her chest. She stepped back from me as if to distance herself. "I believe that's private information," she said.

I decided to try another tactic. "How did they make the Christmas ornaments?"

"We have a volunteer who comes in once a month," she replied. She turned away from me at this point in our brief conversation to look at two patients standing near us in the hallway. "Move along now," she said to them. Then she turned back to me.

"I suggest you speak with our social worker," she said. It was the second time that day someone had suggested I speak with the social worker, so I supposed the social worker must have all the answers to the questions I needed to ask.

Now I stood facing the tree. Behind the tree were tall windows. I could see snow beginning to fall on the ground outside. I cringed, thinking about my long drive home.

I looked around to see if the social worker might be available. She had an office in one of the rooms on the ward. A sign hung next to the door, and I had noticed her speaking with someone only a few minutes before.

Tentatively I stuck my head in her door and cleared my throat. She was sitting behind a large desk that seemed to take up most of the room. She was talking on the phone but waved her hand to indicate I could come in. She put her hand over the receiver.

"Have a seat," she whispered.

I sat down in the only chair that wasn't filled with manila files, books, or papers. As I waited for her to finish her conversation, I looked around. A poster tacked up behind the desk depicted two college-age students drinking soda and smiling.

"Just say NO" was what the poster read. Instinctively I looked down at my watch. I wondered when I could start back home and what the road conditions would be like then. I was still driving a rental car and somewhat skittish about driving because of the recent accident. When the woman finished her phone conversation, she leaned across the desk and extended her hand.

"Hello, I'm Karen Daniels," she said. "You're Ben's mother, correct?"

"Yes," I said. Only my voice came out more like a squeak. "I wanted to talk with you about what programs are available for him since he's going to be leaving the hospital soon."

"Yes," she said. She began sorting through the papers on her desk. Finally she found what she was looking for. She opened a file and looked through the contents. I shifted in my seat and waited. It seemed that all I did in this hospital was wait to see what would happen next.

Karen Daniels looked up again. "It appears that Ben's insurance covers up to 21 days of primary care, which means he will be released next Wednesday," she told me.

"Good Lord, that's soon," I gasped. "Is that enough time?" I asked. "I don't mean to be pushy, but he tried to kill himself. It hardly seems as if he's been here long enough to make a difference."

"That is the amount of time allocated by his insurance company for this kind of treatment," she said. She looked through another file. "It says here that he's been treated for bipolar disorder and has a prescription to take with him when he leaves." She smiled brightly. "Everything seems to be in order."

"Wait a minute!" I said. "You can't just dismiss him like that. What happens next?"

"We have an on-site day program that you can enroll him in if you'd like," she said. He would need to be here at eight in the morning, and someone would have to pick him up by two in the afternoon." She passed a pink photocopied brochure across the desk.

"The main number is listed on the bottom of this flyer if you're interested," she said.

"Does insurance cover this?" I asked.

"You'll have to check with your carrier," she said. "But I believe that most companies will pay a portion of the cost, once you have met the deductible."

"Are you telling me there aren't any other alternatives before we send him back into society again? Something like a halfway house?" I asked.

"Is he alcoholic?" she asked. "There are several halfway houses in the city that are set up to handle addiction-related —" I cut her off in mid-sentence.

"He's not an alcoholic, dammit!" I pushed my chair back and stood up.

"Calm down," she suggested. She motioned me to sit back down. I did, but I was shaky and ready to cry.

"Can't he go home with you?" she asked.

I put my head in my hands and gave a great sigh. "I don't know," I said.

I was remembering the conversation that had taken place between me and Evelyn earlier that morning. She did not want me to bring Ben to her house; not with Mickey there.

She was afraid that Ben might do something to hurt Mickey. We had quarreled about it.

"I live here, remember?" I said. We were sitting across from each other at the dining-room table. "What am I supposed to do with him?"

"Aren't there programs for people like him?" she asked. At this point Evelyn got up from the table and went into the next room. I could hear her rummaging around before she came back and sat down. She dropped a telephone book onto the table. It hit with a thump, spilling my coffee. She sat down and lit a cigarette.

"What's that for?" I asked her.

"It's your resource," she said. She blew a smoke ring at me. "Look up rehab programs. There's got to be someplace where you can send him. They can't just expect you to take him home, especially after what's happened," she said.

And so I looked in the yellow pages, but there seemed to be nothing available for people like my Ben. I made several phone calls that morning, finally finding one facility in the Washington, D.C., area. The people were very nice, but the place was full and there weren't any vacancies for three months. Of course they said they would be happy to put Ben on a waiting list. I told Evelyn as much, but she didn't take the news very well at all. I ended up spending the entire morning on the phone, and Evelyn must have smoked a pack of cigarettes.

"There are no resources, Evelyn," I said.

"Can't he stay with one of his friends?" she asked.

By noon the dining room table was covered with my notes, phone numbers, lists of things to do, an ashtray full of cigarette butts, a couple of empty bottles of soda, and half of an untouched sandwich. Evelyn and I had argued back and forth, getting nowhere. Finally she had asked me to please look a little further. After all, she had her son to think about, too.

"Why don't you talk with the social worker at the hospital?" she suggested. "The social worker should know all about this kind of thing," she added confidently.

So, there I sat, my head in my hands, not knowing what to do, with the social worker named Karen Daniels waiting for me to say something. At that moment I felt as if maybe I should just join Ben in the hospital. There seemed to be no place else to go.

"Miss, are you all right?" Karen Daniels asked me.

I looked up and rubbed my eyes. "I'm sorry," I said. "It's been a long day, and I'm worried. It's snowing hard, and I need to be going home." I pushed my chair back and rose to leave. Karen Daniels stood up with me and leaned across her desk to shake hands.

"Sorry I couldn't be of more help," she said.

"Where do people go who don't have families to go home to?" I asked her suddenly.

There was a long pause before she replied.

"They live on the street," she said.

December 30, 1999

I awoke to the sun streaming in my window. The panes of glass were frosted, but I could see it was going to be a pleasant day. Today I would be bringing Ben back here with me. Evelyn and I had finally come to an agreement that he could stay at the house for the time being. If anything happened that she felt would compromise Mickey's welfare, I would look for other arrangements for Ben. In the meantime, I was hopeful it would work out for everyone concerned.

Evelyn and I had cleared out a space in the attic where Ben could sleep. The ceiling sloped, and it was difficult to stand up in some places, but the window on one end let in enough light, so at least it wasn't gloomy. We had dragged a mattress up the stairs the night before, and I had made up the bed with some linen I'd saved. Evelyn supplied two pillows and an electric blanket. The room wasn't great. It was a temporary solution for January when the temperatures could go down below zero. It was also better than nothing.

I got dressed and made coffee in my studio down the hall from my bedroom. The attic stairs were right behind a door there, which was one of the reasons we'd settled on the attic. There was a new rule in place, however: Mickey was not allowed anywhere on the third floor, and Ben wasn't allowed downstairs when Mickey was home. It wasn't a perfect arrangement, but it would work for the time being.

I knew that Evelyn would be getting Mickey off to school, and I wanted to get out of the house before there was a scene between them. There almost always seemed to be a problem getting Mickey out the door. He would forget one thing or another; this morning I could hear them arguing about his socks. Apparently he couldn't find them, and Evelyn was probably searching through stacks of clothes that had been piling up in the laundry room. I gingerly made my way down the stairs, hoping to avoid them and the latest skirmish. Instead I found Mickey at the bottom of the stairs. I gently pushed him out of my way. "Sorry," I whispered. He shrugged and rolled his eyes. I liked this kid.

"You should have sorted through your clothes last night," Evelyn called from the laundry room.

Mickey didn't say a word, just kept standing there. He shrugged his shoulders again and darted a glance at me as if to say "I give up already!" Instead I shouted back to her, "I'm leaving for work. Don't forget, I'm bringing Ben home tonight." I didn't wait around for her reply; I was out the door. It took 30 minutes to drive into Baltimore. I was glad to have some peace and quiet for a change.

It had snowed a couple of days before, so the countryside was picture-perfect. Off in the distance I could see tiny farmhouses and barns surrounded by what seemed to be miles of white fences. I was driving by the luxurious horse farms of northern Baltimore County. Occasionally I saw a horse or two standing in the distant snowy fields. Those thoroughbreds didn't have a care in the world. What I wouldn't give to be out there right now, painting that landscape.

"Good lord, I'm losing it!" I suddenly thought. I had started to daydream, something that was happening more often these days. Truth was, I wasn't just worried about Ben I was concerned about myself. I felt on the verge of tears over minutiae: Had I left a candle burning somewhere? What was the phone number of Dr. Such and Such? Where were my car keys?

Now I forced myself to concentrate on the road, but I also started to wonder how I was going to pay for everything. How much was Ben's prescription going to cost? I began to mentally add up my income for the past month, stopped, caught myself, and remembered I was driving into Baltimore. I drove in this fashion, remembering details, and then realizing I was on Route 83 proceeding south more or less the entire way to work.

It was Thursday. My first client was Gertrude. I exited at Jones Falls Expressway and drove through Gertrude's neighborhood. It was beautiful, as always, as if a giant had frosted houses, trees, and ponds with thick, white icing. Snow covered everything, even the streets. The houses looked warm and cozy, no one was outside today. I imagined everyone tucked in somewhere nice, sipping hot chocolate. For once, I was grateful I wasn't one of *them*.

I liked my job. I enjoyed the diversity of working for different facilities. Gertrude was my only private client; I visited her twice a week. I had finally adjusted to her home environment and was beginning to feel comfortable around her entire family. Not only did Gertrude live with her son and daughter-in-law, but two granddaughters lived there as well, along with the other mother-in-law, Irene. Irene lived at the other end of the same hallway as Gertrude. She looked a lot like a sweet grandmother, but she could swear like a sailor under duress, whether actual or perceived. There was only one other detail about Irene that was pertinent to me: She hated Gertrude.

Because the streets hadn't been plowed, it was difficult to negotiate the hill, so I pulled my car into the alley behind the house. The alley seemed to be the only place in the whole area that had been dug out. From the driveway, a tiny trail led up to the back door. This path was about a shovel's width and liberally dusted with rock salt. It crunched underfoot as I walked.

I was silently congratulating myself about my idea to leave all the art supplies here at the house. I had stashed everything in Gertrude's dresser drawers, what she called her cupboard. Now I had my hands free, able to negotiate the little path without endangering myself — and I wouldn't have to haul the art box all the way upstairs. Irene met me at the door, wearing an apron over a hot pink gym suit. I could see past her into the kitchen. There was a large mixing bowl on the table, and wonderful aromas were coming from the oven. My stomach began to growl, and Irene must have sensed this.

"I ain't giving out nothing this morning," she said. "That cake is for the party tonight."

"That's wonderful," I said.

Irene stepped back into the kitchen while I remained in the hall. "Don't give me your patronizing crap," she replied. "I still don't see why they bother having someone like you come here and paint with that invalid upstairs! It's a waste of good money if you ask me." Irene picked up the mixing bowl and held it out for me to inspect.

"I keep up my end," she said.

"Yes, well, it's been nice talking with you, but I'm really here to see Gertrude." I started to move toward the stairs. I was halfway up to the landing when Irene shouted something I couldn't understand. It sounded like "The letter leads the dog."

(I found out later that she had said "Don't let her feed that dog.")

"Thank you," I replied.

Gertrude's door was ajar, a good sign. That meant she was awake and possibly dressed.

I pushed it the rest of the way open and entered her room. Gertrude was sitting facing the window, her back to me. She was wearing a faded blue housecoat, her hair in a little cap. The window shade had been raised halfway and was bathing the little room in light. She turned and smiled when she saw me.

"Come in, come right in," she said. "I've been waiting for you all morning."

She was sitting in her new wheelchair. She could still walk, but the Professor had insisted on getting the wheelchair. He was worried she might fall and break a hip. The Mrs. had researched support systems on the internet that would make life easier for a disabled person, and for them. It seemed obvious they had put a lot of thought into her quality of life. I had been hired right before Thanksgiving, and this wheelchair arrived just in time for Christmas.

I pulled open the top dresser drawer, expecting to find the watercolor paper and paint, but it wasn't there. Instead, there were stacks of neatly folded underwear, stockings, and a large bunch of grapes. I picked up the grapes. Frowning, I turned to Gertrude. I held the grapes up to show her.

"What are these doing in your drawers?" I asked.

"I'm saving them," she said.

I decided not to get into it. Instead I asked her where she'd put the paint and paper.

Gertrude pointed to the top of the other dresser. There were the paper, two brushes, and a new box of Winsor-Newton watercolors. I walked over to the dresser and opened the beautiful box, filled with 12 plump, pristine dollops of color. I was dumbstruck while I held it. I had always wanted one.

"Did they get the right thing?" Gertrude asked.

I held the box lovingly in my hands and looked up. "It's beautiful, the most expensive paint money can buy," I said. "You're a lucky woman."

Gertrude frowned slightly at my remarks and patted the metal folding chair by the card table — my chair. Gertrude sat on one side facing the window, and I sat on the other side. Once I had taken my seat, she took the paint box from me and placed it in front of her.

"Life is short, dearie. Be sure to make the most of it," she said.

Ignoring her comment, I laid a piece of watercolor paper down on the table. "What do you want to paint today?" I asked.

"I don't want to paint," she said.

"What do you want to do?" I asked. It seemed like a reasonable request, especially since I already knew she had been depressed. I waited in the silence that followed. It was so quiet that I could hear Irene walking around downstairs.

"I want to be young again," she finally said.

I leaned over, picked up one of the paintbrushes, and placed it in her hand. "Let's pretend you're nine years old," I said. "Tell me what your life was like then."

She thought a moment. "It was nineteen-eighteen," she said. "I remember when my father died. A lot of people died from the flu that year. My mother had him laid out on our dining-room table. There were flowers all around. On the day of the funeral she asked me to go down the street to get a shirt she had had starched at the cleaners. You see, my father only had the one white shirt, and Momma wanted to have him buried in it."

Inwardly I groaned. This was not the conversation I had envisioned between us. I worried that her talking like this was only going to make things worse, not better. Inadvertently, she had reminded me of Ben, how close we had come to death only a few weeks earlier. She kept talking, though, and I had to listen. The Professor was paying me.

"I was scared of the man who owned the cleaners," she went on. "His name was Mr. Chim. He didn't speak very good English either, and I never could understand what he was saying. This particular day when I went in to fetch my father's shirt, he wanted me to spell out my last name. Then he kept repeating the letters over and over, but he didn't get my last name right, and I thought he was telling me to go to hell."

"What letters did he repeat?" I asked.

"H, E, L, L,... O!" she said. "H, E, L, L, O!" Gertrude threw back her head and began laughing. She pulled a tissue from under her sleeve and blew her nose before she looked at me again and smiled.

"After he gave me the shirt, I ran all the way home crying. Poor Momma had to explain to me that old Mr. Chim just couldn't spell," she said.

After that, I was able to sketch a street from her hometown that came out of a book she owned titled *Pittsburgh*. There were many black-and-white photographs of Pittsburgh taken during the 1920s. Gertrude happily pointed out all the landmarks she remembered, finally showing me a picture of the street where she remembered growing up. It was the same street that the cathedral she always talked about was on.

"Here it is!" she exclaimed, "but it looks different now of course." You know I'm going back there someday. Painting and talking with you is nice, but I won't be around here for long. Time can get away from you sometimes," she said.

She was right about the time. I looked down at my watch. It was almost 12:30p.m., and I needed to go. I picked up the watercolor we'd started, along with the paint box and put them back in the dresser drawer. Then I picked up the bunch of grapes I'd left on top of the dresser to take back downstairs.

I turned around to say good-bye and there was Gertrude holding her arms open wide.

"Give me a hug good-bye," she said.

I leaned down and touched my cheek to hers. "I'll be back soon," I said, and then I turned to leave. I didn't see Irene on my way out, but I could hear her moving around below in the family room in the basement of the house.

"Good-bye," I yelled to no one in particular. Nobody answered. So I left the same way I had come in, empty-handed.

Chapter 10

February 15, 2000

It was overcast when I went outside to warm up my car. I could already smell snow in the air even though the weather forecasters hadn't predicted it until later in the day.

It was the gloomy, gray kind of Baltimore day that no one can really appreciate or understand unless they have lived in the area for a long time. Gray comes with winter here, and eventually you have to learn to live with it.

"Like it or lump it," Gertrude says.

As for me, I was lumping it. I had gotten the door open easily, but the car didn't start right up. It sputtered for a while. I was worried; I couldn't afford to lose another day of work. Between the weather and all the driving I had done lately, I was in the hole financially. While I sat waiting for the engine to turn over, it occurred to me that it was crazy to live this far away from the city. It had seemed like a good idea at the time I moved, but my life had changed radically since then.

For one thing, I had been driving Ben to and from the outpatient treatment program at the hospital. It meant that I had to get up earlier every morning and interrupt my day to pick him up. It was difficult knowing exactly what to do with him afterward, since I usually had one more dementia class to teach in the afternoon. Ben was still not ready to come along with me as a volunteer, either. We finally decided that he could wait for me in the lobby at the hospital until I was done. I hated leaving him there. He was still unpredictable, and I didn't know what he might do. We had gone back and forth about another solution for the last couple of days. Then this morning he had asked me if he could just stay home.

"I'm tired, Mom," he complained.

This morning I had climbed up the back stairs to the attic and found him sleeping under a pile of blankets. The room was chilly; it made me shiver. I wished I had never moved out of my apartment back in town. I leaned down and shook him gently. He rolled over and moaned when he saw me.

"Leave me alone," he said.

"Come on, Ben, get up," I implored.

"I hate going to that place," he said. "Most of the people who go there are either nuts or retarded or something!"

I sat down on the mattress next to him, pulling one of the blankets off the top of the pile to wrap around me for warmth. Once my eyes adjusted to the dark, I could see my breath.

It was a low point for me to think that this was the best I could do for my son. Suddenly it came over me that I was a failure as a human being, as a mother. Hot tears started to well up in my eyes and I was grateful for the darkness so he wouldn't see.

"Got any suggestions?" I asked, turning my face away from him.

Ben pulled the covers down, exposing only his face. "I want to paint," he replied.

I looked around the attic. "Here?" I asked.

"Last time I looked, you had a studio right down those stairs. There's plenty of paint, too," he said. "I can paint while you're at work."

All I could do was nod my head in agreement. Why hadn't I thought of that in the first place? "What are you going to paint?" I asked. He shrugged his shoulders.

"Let's get up then," I suggested. "I'm going down to start up the car before I go to work. You get dressed and pour yourself a cup of coffee while I'm outside. OK?" He nodded and smiled at me. After that, I left him to get dressed. I quickly ran down the two flights of stairs leading out to the driveway.

The car finally started up, and I let out my breath in relief. Ben could stay here during the day. I liked the idea. What harm could he cause anyone in the empty house? Certainly Evelyn would allow him kitchen privileges during the day while Mickey was at school. Maybe I should tell Evelyn about these new changes in plans. I didn't want her running around the house after she'd gotten out of the shower or something, not with Ben there.

Satisfied that the car would get me into town, I turned it off. I loved the old thing, a little red Mazda convertible. I didn't need to leave the car on long to keep the heater running, because it worked fine, but on really cold days like this, I kept an old wool blanket in the passenger seat. Throwing the blanket over my lap kept the worst of the cold off my legs, but I was always glad when it got to be spring.

Getting out, I slammed the door, noticing how much better it worked since the repair shop had fixed it. I stamped my way through a snow bank to the house and knocked the snow off my boots by the back door. Once inside, I couldn't help but notice the firewood that Lewis's friend had neatly stacked at the back of the porch. It had certainly come in handy with all the cold weather we'd had lately. There is nothing worse than bringing in wood with snow all over it. It's almost impossible to start a fire with wet wood. I rubbed my hands together, warming them before going to find Evelyn.

She didn't look up as I walked into the kitchen. Evelyn was leaning over the counter, examining her face in the mirror she was holding and drinking a diet Coke. Next to her a cigarette lay smoldering in the ashtray, quite forgotten. It was burning down to a long ash.

"What?" she said.

I pulled a stool over to the other side of the counter so I'd be facing her. Actually, I was facing the back side of Evelyn's mirror, which rather defeated my purpose of a one-on-one conversation, but I went ahead and told her my idea anyway. Now I had her immediate attention.

She put the mirror down, and then reached around behind her. What she found was a filter attached to an ash. This she ground out rather unceremoniously in the ashtray, all the while looking around, feeling her pockets, and looking for her cigarette pack. I hastily pulled two cigarettes out of my pack of Marlboros, knowing it wasn't her brand, offering her one.

"Thanks," she said, eyeing me.

"Well, what do you think of our idea?" I asked.

"I don't think it's going to work," she said. "What happened to the daycare thing he was going to?"

"He told me that he hates it, says that it's a bunch of lunatics. He feels out of place there," I said. Then as an afterthought, "It's been hard on me, too, with all the driving back and forth."

Evelyn leaned closer to me across the counter where we were sitting. It seemed as if she had something important to say. I held my breath, expecting the worst: Either she wasn't going to go for it or ask me to find another place to live. Instead she surprised me.

"You'll have to pay more rent while he's here then," was what she said.

"I don't see how I can," I whined. "Right now I'm pretty strapped. I've also got to start making his child support payments."

Sometimes Evelyn had more imagination than I did. What she told me next was that I would have to resolve my personal relationship with the material world. She actually said, "You need to get flat about money."

"What are you getting at?" I asked. Suddenly my brains had turned to blubber.

"Let me ask you a question," she said. "Didn't you just get some money from the insurance on your car accident?"

"Yep, but I've already spent it."

"That statement alone serves as an excellent example of your dysfunction," she explained. I must have looked confused, because Evelyn kept talking. She told me that I needed to raise rates for my services and get all the facilities to pay me in advance. Finally she said, "You need to call in your resources."

"I hate it when you use that word," I said. "What's that supposed to mean?"

Evelyn looked at me as if I were hopelessly stupid. "Ask the Professor for an advance so you can afford your life!" she commanded. "He already knows you're not going anywhere with a six-month contract. Besides, he's got plenty of dough, doesn't he?"

"I can't ask him that!" I gasped.

"And that's exactly why you have issues with money," she said.

There was no time for a rebuttal. Behind Evelyn I could see the kitchen clock; it was nearly 9:00 a.m. I had to get going soon or I'd be late. "Oh my," I exclaimed and jumped up. "I've got to get to work!"

Evelyn picked the mirror up, smiled back into it, and continued to examine her face. The entire time her attention seemed to be focused more on herself than on me, but she spoke again. While she talked, she gazed at her reflection.

"Think about what I've told you," she said.

"I know Evelyn," I said. "I will."

It seemed clear she wanted me to have a better quality of life, just as Gertrude's family wanted the best for her. I pondered this as I walked across the kitchen that morning. I wondered how anyone else could possibly determine the best thing for me. I shook my head with confusion as I mounted the stairs.

"How dare she tell me what to do?" I thought.

Once again I ran up the stairs to let Ben know he could stay at home. When I walked into the studio he was already dressed, wearing an old sweat shirt and a pair of warm-up pants. The sweat shirt had two holes in the front, and his feet were bare. He was standing in front of an old wooden easel where he had propped up a large canvas.

"You look like an old hippie," I commented.

He laughed at this. "It's all I could find to wear," he said.

"Oh yeah," I replied. I kept forgetting we'd left most of his stuff in Florida. "I need to take you clothes shopping," I said.

He nodded in agreement. "I need snow boots, too," he said.

I didn't know how I was going to take him shopping, but I decided not to tell him that right now. Something might work out in the meantime, I just didn't know what. I thought about what Evelyn had said earlier, then I thought about what the Professor would say if I asked him to give me money — money that I hadn't earned yet.

Ben interrupted my thoughts. "What were you thinking just then?" he asked.

"How I wish we were somewhere warm," I lied.

"I'll paint you a beach!" he said.

"That's a great idea," I said. I'm leaving for work in about five minutes, but I should be home around 4:30. I hope to make it back before it snows again."

"I'll be right here," he said. "I can't go very far without boots now, can I?"

I looked down at his bare feet and sighed. Ben grabbed my shoulder. "It's all right Mom," he said.

"Thanks, but remember not to cook anything in the kitchen. Just make a sandwich today, OK?" I asked. "We'll take this one step at a time."

He nodded. "Gotcha," he replied.

Back outside it was getting colder, clouds were building up, and the front was coming in. I got into my car and pulled the blanket over my legs. The car started up on the first try, and I carefully backed down the long driveway. It was slick and treacherous. The snow was packed down; we hadn't shoveled out from the last storm. For some reason or another, it made me laugh. I was definitely going to have to talk with Evelyn about our shoveling resources. If Lewis was still around, maybe he could help.

The first stop that day was at a retirement community. I worked at the healthcare center there with a group of very low-functioning residents. We had stuffed large paper bags with newspaper the week before, and then painted them completely white. My idea was to stack three of them, adding an old hat at the top to make snowmen. The activity assistant had promised me she would find old hats for today's class.

I entered the facility through large front doors that automatically opened, allowing me hands-free entry into the building. This was welcome, because I was hauling a large box of paints and assorted crafts on a luggage carrier. I'd also brought along scissors, paper, glitter, and white glue in an attempt to be prepared in case the activity staff wasn't. One of the mottos among those of us who service nursing facilities is "Be prepared for anything." In that respect I guess you could say I had the same principles as a Girl Scout.

Waiting in the reception area was a group of old ladies dressed for cold weather.

They were fussing with hats, scarves, and gloves and looked as if they were going someplace special. One or two carried handbags, some had wooden canes, while others pushed wire baskets on wheels.

"We're going grocery shopping," one said as I walked by. I stopped just long enough to inspect the group.

"But you're all dressed up," I said.

"We don't get out much," she explained. Several of her companions laughed at the remark.

"Stay warm," I advised them.

I kept moving with my art supplies in tow and turned a corner to get on the elevator that would take me up to the dreaded fourth floor. Most of the healthier, independent residents had an aversion to the healthcare center located there. They called it "death row." When I got off the elevator, I turned and walked down the length of the hall to the resident's dining area. It was a large, bright room that served part-time as a dining room and the activity room in between meals. As a result of the dual function, there always seemed to be leftover food stuck to tables and the floor. Occasionally I had found bananas or packages of dried cereal hidden behind the curtains. Many of the residents pocketed sugar packets and other supplies that they squirreled away in their rooms. This was not because they didn't get enough to eat; it was because they had lived through the Depression, then the war. They had been taught to save everything, and they did.

Three tables were pushed together and covered with newspaper. Around these tables the activity assistant, Judy, had situated seven individuals. All but one rode in a wheelchair. Judy had left space between each wheelchair so that I could squeeze in between them while we painted. I didn't have my own assistant then, so it would be just Judy and me working with the group. And bless their hearts, the residents all looked up expectantly, happy to see me. I would be remiss not to admit that they brightened my spirits most of the time. First I said hello to everyone, then started getting paint out of the box, moving around the tables as I did so, touching their shoulders, giving hugs from behind. I spoke to Judy as I was doing this. She had been working in the healthcare center for only a couple of weeks.

'Where's Clara today?" I asked.

"I decided not to bring her. She never paints or anything, so I left her in her room," Judy explained.

I stopped what I was doing. I could feel the heat rise up in my face in response to her statement. Around the table my seven darlings looked from me to Judy in great expectation. Judy stood twisting her hands together, but she didn't move an inch from where she stood.

"Go get her," I said.

"She don't paint," she said again.

"I'm not asking, I'm telling you," I said. "Clara has been a part of this class for the last six months."

Judy motioned for me to follow her into the hallway. Once we were out of range from the others, she began telling me that poor old Clara was unable to speak, couldn't feed herself, and would only be in the way.

"She ain't right," Judy said.

"I know all that, but I happen to believe that she *is* all right. She just doesn't communicate like you or me. And more so, I think she's trapped in her body with no way out," I said.

After hearing me out, Judy huffed off down the hall like a child who had been reprimanded. Two minutes later, she was back in the dining room, pushing Clara.

"You can wheel her over there at the head of the table," I said. "She can see better there."

"I can't stay the entire time," Judy said suddenly.

"Why not?" I asked.

"I've got to transport a new resident up to her room. It's her first day," she said.

"Why don't you bring her in here with us?" I suggested. "She'll get a chance to meet everyone."

Judy left, and I gave one of the stuffed grocery bags to each person seated around the tables, then handed out paintbrushes as well. At first glance, I didn't see any hats, so I made a mental note to ask Judy when she got back. We were going to create snowmen and make an exhibit out in the hall today, and the residents were excited. Someone had remembered to save two bags of fake snow left over from Christmas. I intended to roll it out around the bottom of the snowmen. This morning it was slow going, working alone. One resident, Charles was painting the inside of a plastic cup instead of the bag.

"Let's stay on purpose, Charles," I told him gently. He looked up and smiled at me.

It was easy to see he enjoyed the attention. I put the paintbrush back in his hand, showing him how to hold it and paint. Finally he got the hang of it. I could tell he was pleased with himself, too.

"Look," he said. "It's Frosty!"

It took about ten minutes to get them all actively engaged with the paint and the stuffed bags. I looked up for a moment to take a breath. It's not easy to be with seven or eight disabled individuals by yourself and not get tired. They require lots of energy. Today I felt exhausted. Outside the dining room I could hear someone shouting and crying. The commotion seemed to be getting louder, so I left the class briefly to see what was going on. Looking down the hall, I could see Judy pushing a woman in a wheelchair toward me. The lady was kept in the chair by a restraint that looked a lot like a cushion that had been strapped into place in front of her. As Judy approached, I could see the lady trying to disengage herself from the contraption by yanking at it. She was crying inconsolably. Judy stopped pushing the lady, breathless.

"I can't get her to stop crying," she groaned. "What am I going to do now?"

"What's her name?" I asked.

"Mrs. Thompson," Judy said.

I squatted down so that I was at eye level with Mrs. Thompson. She had started to rub her eyes, and they were all puffy and red. The only makeup she wore was rouge, and that was now running down both sides of her face, leaving two streaks. I looked up at Judy.

"I don't suppose you remembered to get those hats for today did you?" I asked her.

Judy gave me a blank look. "I guess I forgot," she said.

"Never mind, let's bring this one into the dining room. Maybe we can distract her," I suggested.

I placed both my hands over Mrs. Thompson's hands and smiled at her. Instead of smiling back, she slapped me, sending me reeling backward. I caught myself just before hitting the floor. "Are you OK?" Judy asked. She looked panic-stricken. There wasn't time to console her; we needed to move Mrs. Thompson out of the hall in a hurry. I waved Judy off, pointing in the direction of the dining room. Catching my breath, I found my voice again.

"Move it! I mean her," I said.

While Judy and I had been wrestling with Mrs. Thompson in the hall, my painting class had become completely chaotic in the dining room. They had stopped painting and were listening. Apparently they had heard everything that had been going on in the hall. A resident named Sue said, "I heard every word perfectly!" She pulled a hearing aid out of her ear and turned it over to look closer at it. "This thing works pretty darn good when I use it," she exclaimed.

Meanwhile Judy wheeled Mrs. Thompson in to the dining room, but now the new arrival had started to cry again, only louder. Worse still, her crying was juxtaposed between great big sobs. She kept yelling that she wanted to go home.

"Take me home," she screamed, clawing at her face with her hands.

I realized much too late that it had been a mistake to try to include Mrs. Thompson in with the art therapy class. It was as if the entire room had gone straight to hell. Several of my painters had also started to cry. Mrs. Thompson served to remind them that they wanted to go home, too. I don't remember how long the chaos went on, but out of the blue someone started to sing "God Bless America." Surprised, I looked around and got the shock of my life.

It was Clara singing. Clara, who hadn't spoken a word for months, who couldn't even feed herself. Clara was the one whom everyone considered just short of a vegetable. She was singing with a deep tenor voice.

"Land that I love ... Stand beside her... and guide her... through the night, with the light from above ..."

One by one we all began to sing with her. What else could we do? If there was a second verse, none of us could remember it, so we all sang the same verse several times over again. Even poor Mrs. Thompson sang. Through the act of singing she had forgotten all about herself or wanting to go home, and blessedly so had the others.

It was noon by the time I got out of the building that day, and the sky was starting to spit snow. It was coming down lightly as I made my way across the parking lot. I got back into my car and turned on the ignition so I could run the heater. It was freezing outside. I looked out through the window while I considered making a call to the Professor. It was lunchtime, and I might just find him available in his office. I was too scared to talk to him in person. Maybe this was a mistake; perhaps I was being too forward? After sitting there for another five minutes, I decided to go ahead and ask him for the money. I did some calculating while I sat in the car, figuring an extra thousand dollars would be enough. If he agreed, the Professor would be consenting to pay me in advance for the next two months. I picked up my cell phone, dialed his number at the university, thought better of it, and then quickly hung up. I did this several times while I sat there, running the car with the heat on full-blast.

Meanwhile the snow continued to come down. It had started to stick to the sidewalks leading up to the building. I watched two people walking around the outside of the building with their heads turned down. One of them was hurriedly wrapping a scarf around her neck while she walked. It occurred to me as I watched them that I would have to cancel my afternoon classes. All the more reason then to call the Professor I told myself. I took a deep breath and dialed his number again. The phone rang several times, but this time he answered. I started out by telling him it was me.

"Did you just call?" he asked.

"Oh, yes sir," I said breathlessly. "But I must be in a bad cell, lost the connection you know."

"Yes," he said. "I'm getting ready to go into a meeting right now, only have a couple of minutes to talk. What can I do for you?"

"I called to ask a favor of you, sir," I replied.

"And that is?"

'Well, I believe you know my son has been in the hospital; there's been a lot of medical expenses I hadn't counted on, and I was wondering if it was possible to have you pay me a bit in advance?" I asked. When he didn't say anything, I stopped talking. On his end I could hear a door being closed in the background.

"Just a minute," he said. Now I could hear him saying something, but he must have held his hand over the receiver because the sound was muffled. He seemed to be having a conversation with somebody else. My heart was in my throat. I sat there silently cursing Evelyn for getting me into this in the first place. Finally he got back on the phone.

"Sorry," he said. "What were you saying?" I couldn't believe it. I was going to have to ask him all over again. This time I decided to be more direct.

"I need to ask for a thousand-dollar advance covering the next two months," I blurted out.

"Yes," he said. "I understand that your son has been in the hospital recently. Sorry to hear that." As the Professor talked, I literally held my breath. I squeezed my eyes shut and asked again.

"Is it possible to get paid in advance?" A long silence followed. I held my little phone closer to my ear hoping that I hadn't lost the connection. If that happened, I would have to call him back and go through this one more time. While I waited, I could hear the Professor eating his lunch. He started to speak, but his words came out in spurts, not sentences. Whatever he was attempting to say was crammed in between his sandwich.

"Sorry, trying to eat what the Mrs. packed for me," he said. Then silence. "It's tuna fish. Wait just a minute." Then silence. "Hold on there, thanks," he said between bites.

I was almost in tears. I had called at the worst time! I was never going to listen to anybody else's advice as long as I lived, that much was certain. "I've got to go now," automatically came out of my mouth."

"I can advance you five hundred dollars," he said.

"Oh thank you, sir," I gasped. "You won't have to worry or anything like that!"

"Worry about what indeed!" he said. "Glad that the Mrs. and I can help. Your check will be waiting the next time you see my mother."

"Thank you again," I said.

"No problem, but I really have to go now," the Professor said. I collapsed back in my seat and watched the snow come down. I hadn't gotten the whole thing, but I had done it!

I'd been able to get beyond my considerations and ask for

what I needed. At any rate, I felt encouraged. I remembered Clara singing earlier, how she had also done something remarkable, quite out of the ordinary. If Clara could do it, then so could I, and on this note I vowed never to allow myself to feel like a victim again.

I remained in this positive state of mind all the way home. I arrived in time to negotiate the driveway, aiming for the ruts that had already been worn into the gravel. There wasn't so much snow that I'd have to back down several times before getting to the top. I saw that Evelyn's car was still parked there, too, which meant she hadn't gone to pick up Mickey yet. This was good because I was eager to tell her my news. I ran into the house, stopping briefly to remove my boots on the back porch. Inside Evelyn was sitting in front of the fireplace sorting through the mail.

"Did you get anything interesting?" I asked. I dropped down onto the couch next to her.

On the coffee table in front of her was a stack of letters and bills. She stopped in the middle of opening one with her fingernail, and then looked over at me. Instead of saying anything, Evelyn simply handed me a bill from the gas and electric company. I looked at it, noting that it was dated from January.

"It's over a thousand dollars!" she exclaimed. Immediately my heart sank. My good news would pale in comparison, but I went ahead and told her that the Professor had given me an advance for five hundred dollars.

"Good," she said. "Now you can pay for your half of the heating bill."

Chapter 11

May 7, 2000

I was suddenly awake, hearing quite plainly an opera from above me. I listened briefly, long enough to realize the words were all in Italian: *l'aurora, di bianco vestita, gia luscious dischiude al gran sol...* . I looked out the window and had to think for a minute where I was. Waking up can sometimes be confusing when you move all the time or when you are traveling; with me it had been the former.

I remembered that I was in my own bedroom, in the new apartment, in a little suburb just outside of Baltimore. I had been living in the apartment for the last three months, but I wasn't used to it yet. Sometimes I thought I was still in the country and that when I got out of bed, my old bathroom was still just down the hall. But my life was different than it was before; everything had changed again. There was an apple tree behind my apartment and a little stream just beyond the tree. Behind the tree and the river was a forest where birds were singing. I turned over in my bed and listened to the Italian songs from above. *Ove tu sei nasce l'amor...* (where you are love is born).

The clock radio had come on, interfering with the opera from the neighbor's apartment. The announcer was saying that it was Sunday, 10 o'clock, and the possibility for rain was slim to none. I sat up and turned the radio off. It was time to get up. I tiptoed out into the living room, not sure whether Ben was sleeping or not. His bedroll was stuffed behind the couch, so I assumed that he was at work already. We were roommates now.

After he came home from the hospital, we stayed another six weeks with Evelyn, but the distance from the city was too great, and there was only the one car. Ben had found a job, so I drove him back and forth for a couple of weeks, but that soon got old. I needed to buy him a used car and begin paying off some of the medical bills, too. I needed another source of money, and the solution had been to teach a regular painting class to normal adults as my fund-raising effort. It had been Lewis's idea. I had been lamenting about lack of money, and he had said, "Why don't you teach an independent painting class?"

"Are you crazy?" I had asked him.

"Well, it's something you already know how to do," he explained.

"The last thing I need is one more student, normal or not!" I said. "What do you think I do all week long?"

"What are your other options?" Lewis had asked me.

Of course he was right. I had no other options.

To complicate things, Richard had called and wanted to sign up for art lessons. Apparently Lewis had told him about the class. At first, I had objected. I was worried. He was a married man, and lonely. I knew this because he had driven out to visit me again while I was still living at Evelyn's house, right after the Christmas holidays. That afternoon he had talked about his life and his unhappy marriage. It definitely explained a lot about him, like why he was spending weekends hiking in the country with Lewis and paying random visits to Evelyn and me when he could have been eating brunch at the Hopkins Club back in town.

It sounded as if his wife was lonely, too. She seemed to spend much of her time and Richard's money on facials, clothes, manicures, and visiting her psychiatrist twice a week. Richard told me that she was about as warm and fuzzy as a cold stone. He went into some detail about how she had achieved a type of perfection with the help of several plastic surgeries, but the surgeries had left her with all the allure of an ill-tempered mannequin. They lived in the best part of town, right down the street from the Professor and Gertrude, where all the little ducks and duck mommies hung out around the perfect ponds. What a life!

So he had found out about the painting class from Lewis, and he wanted to sign up. "I'll pay you in advance," he had said. It was a tempting offer, too. He wanted to pay me in advance for the whole season!

"No way, Richard," had been my response.

Sometime the next day Linda Sue called. "I think you should let Richard in the class," she informed me.

"He's unhappily married," I told her. "It will be a disaster."

"I talked with him, he needs a friend," she said.

"I don't need any more friends with problems," I told her.

"All he does is go to work, and then he mulches," she said.

"What are you talking about?" I asked.

"He told me his main satisfaction in his spare time is working in the garden. He ordered ten cubic yards of mulch, and he spends all of his time mulching the flower beds in that huge yard. He's lonely!" she said.

"It's still no!" I said.

"If he pays in advance, you'd have enough money to pay for Ben's car," she said.

"You are so Jewish," I said.

"Be practical," she retorted.

And so in the end I relented and let Richard into the painting class. We had all been painting for a month now. We gathered at the local Starbuck's coffee shop every Sunday and drove together out to the country. I had four students: Jen, a normal college student type; her mother, Carolyn, a recovering alcoholic; Linda Sue, my best friend; and Richard, the unhappily married doctor, my new friend.

The class convened at 1:00 p.m. After we'd bought our coffee, we would decide where to paint. I liked the idea of the group making the decision. It was the best way for me to feel that I was just along for the ride and for them to begin to participate with one another.

I was moving slowly this morning though, mostly because it seemed hot already, even though it was only May. I opened the bedroom window to see how hot it really was. I could hear the hum of a million bugs outside. I slammed the window shut and went into my little kitchen to start the coffee. By the time I had showered, dressed, and had eaten a piece of toast, it was nearly 12:45p.m. I hurried out the door, knowing full well that I would be about five minutes late and probably the last one there. I was right about both: My class was waiting outside in the parking lot. They had gathered in a tight huddle, and everybody waved as I maneuvered my car behind them.

Hot air rose up from the pavement and met me head-on when I climbed out of my car. It was oppressive. I was beginning to believe this class had been a bad idea. I would never listen to anyone else's advice again, most certainly not Lewis's. Now I was stuck performing as an art instructor for the next two hours, and worse, for the next two months! I was sorry that I needed the money.

Richard jaunted across the parking lot as I was unloading my car. He was dressed like he was going on some kind of safari, complete with a backpack and a straw hat cocked to one side. He carried a folding chair in one hand, his French easel and paints in the other. Richard was smiling, happy to see me. I, on the other hand, was not happy to see anyone that day. I felt as if I was always in charge, that the burden of responsibility rested with me. Mostly I felt like a rundown entertainer, now acting in commercials instead of movies. I was tired of being an artist, and I wanted to go home.

"Great to see you!" he called.

"Same," I responded.

Richard stopped just short of running into my car. He dropped all his gear on the pavement and leaned closer as if to hug me. I saw the inevitable and turned to one side just in time to avoid close personal contact. Instead, he ended up giving me a wet kiss on the side of my cheek.

"Knock it off, Richard," I said. "I'm your art teacher, not your girlfriend, remember?" I rubbed his kiss off with the side of my arm.

"I'm just happy to see you," he said.

I could see Jen, her mother, and Linda Sue giggling behind him. "Just tone it down a little. We've got a fan club," I said, nodding my head toward the group. He turned around quickly and then back to me again, realizing that everyone was amused.

"Gosh, sorry," he said.

"I'd like to maintain my professional reputation," I told him. "Where are we going this afternoon?"

Before Richard could say another word, Linda Sue answered for him with a question. She strode over and slapped me on the back. "How do you feel about north Baltimore county?" she asked. "I have a friend who lives down the road from St. James Church in Monkton, and he's got an awesome pond with ducks." "It's a nice drive out to the country," Linda Sue added.

I looked at Richard. "Can we all fit in your car?" I asked.

"Let's go!" he said beckoning to Jen and her mom. And with that we were packing off to the country, all of us, together.

June 18, 2000

The weeks wore on, and my outlook slowly improved in spite of the way I'd initially felt about teaching another painting class just for the money. I began to enjoy interacting with adults whose only impairment was being bored with their lives in a general, sub-clinical kind of way. The five of us talked, and we painted some, too. I found out that Jen's mom had recovered from a bout with cancer earlier that year. We all wanted to know how she had made it through her ordeal.

"One day at a time," she told us. "I learned that from my AA meetings."

Linda Sue hated her entire family. "They just don't get me," she said. "I'm different from them, they're all terrible workaholics."

"Excuse me; don't you receive a nice little stipend every year from a trust fund your mother set up?" I asked. "You don't have any worries."

"It doesn't matter if no one loves you," she replied.

We got to know each other in ways we normally couldn't have in any other context. Was it because we finally got into the right side of our brains by painting together, or were we were just comforted by one another's sadness? Richard was waiting for his wife to get a job, but none of us could see the significance. It was Jen's mom who finally put our queries about his wife to a halt. "More will be revealed," she said knowingly. Further second-hand wisdom from AA, we decided. But we did back off.

One day we had set up our easels in an alley behind some old buildings to paint images of their slow decay. The houses had fascinated me because of their inherent ability to stand for 200 years despite the obvious lack of care. Whoever might have loved and cherished them had forgotten or been busy doing other things.

"It seems like such a waste, not caring about other people or places, like this house," I commented.

It was just the two of us that particular day, Richard and me. Everybody else was on vacation; it was the first time we had ever been alone together. I felt awkward, because to me it seemed more like a date than an art lesson. Richard, however, seemed as if he were light years away. It was hot, and the air was silent and muggy. I was sweating. When he didn't comment, I decided to change the subject.

"I'm going to raise the class tuition," I said. I waited to see if he had heard me or not. When he still didn't respond, I began to worry. Maybe it was a huge mistake coming out here at all, just him and me.

"My wife is still working on her resumé," Richard finally said.

"What are you talking about?" I asked.

"She doesn't have any real experience," he said.

"Then why is she editing her resumé?" I asked. "I mean, it's not like she has to go to work. She enjoys a privileged life, doesn't she?"

"She feels unfulfilled now that the boys are in college," he said.

"What about you?" I asked.

"Oh, I have a good job," he said.

Richard pulled his shoulders back and stretched. He looked at me and then shrugged. "Listen, my wife doesn't really care about me, only my paycheck. I'm the one who is unfulfilled. I want to leave the marriage, have a chance for romance, and then live happily ever afterward." he said.

"You sound like a fairytale," I said, and laughed.

"I'm not joking," he said.

"And you're waiting for her to find a job so you can do this?" I asked.

"Something like that," he grinned.

I started to laugh again. He was making very broad statements and basing his decision on what his wife might or might not do. "What if she doesn't find a job?" I asked. "What if she doesn't want you to leave?"

Richard frowned and put his paintbrush down. He cleared his throat and stretched, but he looked more like a deer staring into the headlights of a truck. He licked his lips several times before he spoke again.

"*When* she finds a job," he corrected me, "I will leave the marriage. I want my life back." "Listen Richard, it's never a good time to leave," I said. "It will seem like a good time, and then it's Mother's Day, or someone's birthday, Christmas, a birth, Cousin Alice breaks her leg, you lose money in the stock market, or whatever. The truth is, it's never a good time to leave if you're waiting for something to happen."

"What would you do if you were me?" he asked.

I hate it when someone asks me a question about what I would or would not do, especially when my answer might influence an outcome that is none of my business. I hesitated, not knowing what to say. *I've put my foot into it this time,* I thought to myself.

"I'd stay married," I said. "I'd advise you to stay married if at all possible. Divorce is the worst thing you can do to yourself and your family, even if your kids are all grown up. Don't leave hoping that the grass is greener somewhere else, or with someone else. It seldom is."

Richard looked forlorn. He stepped back slightly from his canvas and whipped his brush on the side of his jeans. When he looked back at me again, I could tell that the wind had gone out of his sails.

"You're right," he said. "When you don't care about anyone or anything, it's a terrible waste of a life."

"Richard, go home," I said. "Painting class is over for today."

The truth was that I never intended to see him again. I thought a lot about what it had felt like to spend part of an afternoon with him, how comfortable it was just being there, despite the seriousness of our conversation. He had laughed at my jokes, and he was married to someone else. I made a decision after we got into our separate cars to leave: I was going to call him the following week and let him know that I had decided to end the class early. I was going to return the remainder of his tuition and end this strange friendship once and for all. I really was, but that's not what happened.

June 23, 2000

Several days later, two policemen knocked at my apartment door, looking for Ben. They had official papers from Collier County in Naples, Florida. The papers turned out to be a court injunction preventing Ben from visiting his son unless it could be substantiated that he had recovered and was under the care of a doctor. There were several pages of rules to be agreed to and then signed.

After they had gone, I read over all the papers. I was going to need an official doctor's statement about Ben's mental condition. I decided it would be simpler if I called Richard and asked if he would type a letter for me, rather than hunt down all the shrinks who had first seen Ben. After all, Richard probably knew as much about Ben's medical condition as any of them, and he could also use that fancy doctor language to substantiate the facts. So, I called him, and he agreed to write a letter.

"Why don't you come over now?" he asked.

"Are you sure this is a good time? I don't want to interrupt anything," I told him. What I really meant was that I didn't want to run into his wife. He must have sensed my concern because his answer was reassuring.

"My wife is out getting her hair done, and the maids are here cleaning," he said. "It's just me and the dog."

I knew he lived right around the corner from Gertrude, but I had never been on his street, and I was unprepared when I drove around the circular drive leading up to his house. It was a huge mansion, built mostly of gray stone blocks. It rose like a church and was surrounded by lush gardens. At first, I thought I must have gotten the directions wrong, and I was getting ready to leave. But no, the address was correct. Then the front door opened, and Richard came running out. I stepped from my car, looking up at the house. "This is where you live?" I asked. I was incredulous. I knew he was well-off, but I was completely unprepared for the opulence of the house and the grounds. Richard ignored my surprise and grabbed an old bronze handle on the large wooden door. He pulled the door handle with a flourish and stood holding the door open for me.

"This way, madam."

I didn't say anything to him, just pushed by and found myself standing in a vestibule. In front of me was yet another door made of clear leaded glass. It looked like the entrance to the front hallway. Richard squeezed around me and opened the second door.

"Come on in," he said.

Inside, the air was cold in comparison to the summer heat

outside. I was in standing in the middle of a foyer. The floor was made from polished black and white squares of inlaid marble. I saw a harpsichord with a vase of fresh cut flowers placed on top. To one side a spiral staircase rose gracefully. Portraits in gilded frames, probably ancestors, rose along the wall with the stairs. I could hear a vacuum cleaner running somewhere in the distance. The house had a peculiar smell, like old church hymnals and furniture polish.

To the right was a sitting room with a fireplace at one end. Inside this room were pieces of Victorian furniture, two red striped couches facing each other, and more large oil paintings on the walls. To the left was a formal dining room and another fireplace. A huge crystal chandelier hung over the table, on which were placed even more fresh flowers.

I was immobilized. I couldn't find my voice, but I was able to think about Richard in a whole new way. I was standing in the middle of what looked like a perfect and extravagant life. Up until now, I had seen him only out in the countryside, painting, and wearing khakis and old T-shirts with paint on them — just like me. But I wasn't like him. That much was obvious, standing in the foyer that day and smelling church hymnals. He had a family that was still intact. He lived in a mansion in the best part of town where wives got to stay home and take care of their children, where dinner was served in a dining room that could seat 20 people.

He had a picture-perfect life. I couldn't help but compare it to my own. I had worked since I was 15 years old because I had to. I had received a master's degree, but only for the purpose of earning a decent living, not because I was even remotely interested in a career path or because I wasn't "fulfilled." What I had really wanted to do was grow a vegetable garden. Had anyone ever asked me? No. There was never time to think about such nonsense in a life that was all about surviving.

I realized in the foyer that day that I was the one who had been surviving. Even old Gertrude had a family. Families were important; they made all the difference in the world. For years, there had been no one who really cared about me. I started to cry, right there, with the fresh flowers and Richard's ancestors watching me from the stairwell. My shoulders began to shake, and I threw my hands up over my eyes. I was suddenly ashamed to be me. Richard, of course, had no idea what any of this was about. I must have looked crazy.

"What's the matter?" he asked.

"I'm an orphan!" I wailed and burst into fresh tears.

Suddenly his arms were going around me, pulling me close. I looked up to see him crying right along with me. "What are you crying for?" I blubbered.

"I can't stand to see you in pain," he said.

"What possible difference can that make to you?" I asked.

"I love you," he said.

Chapter 12

September 13, 2000

The summer passed rapidly for Ben and me. He was able to get a job early in June as a line cook for a local restaurant. Ben worked part-time at first, and then began adding more hours. I drove him back and forth to work. It was rough sometimes, especially when he closed up late, but I did it. Things were getting better, though. By the time June rolled around, it seemed as if nothing had ever happened at all; then he had another episode. Strange as it sounds, it still took me by surprise. Looking back, I realize I should have seen it coming, but as Gertrude used to say, "Hindsight is always 20/20."

All summer I had had a full schedule of classes in addition to the plein-air class I continued to teach on the weekends. In fact, I had become so busy that my attention was channeled in other directions: mostly on my career. Ben managed his own schedule. Gertrude once asked me, "How do you know there's a train wreck coming?" To which I exclaimed, "I don't know, how?"

"You look up," she said.

Ben had started hallucinating again, so we made another trip to the hospital. It was upsetting, but different. Now he was under the care of two doctors: a psychiatrist and a neurologist. We wouldn't have to spend 12 hours in the emergency room this time. As I drove him to the hospital, I thought how much easier it was going to be. I parked the car in the visitors' lot and looked over at my son. I felt I had the situation under control.

"This is nothing," I said. "Heck, we've been through worse than this!" Ben said nothing, just sat there and shrugged.

All I really wanted for him, for us, was to have a normal life. By this I meant an ordinary kind of life: You went to school, got married, bought a house, had some kids, and then lived happily ever after. Gertrude tells me that when life happens, it is usually haphazard. "God's got a plan, but it's a secret," she said.

I put my hand on Ben's shoulder. I wanted to say something more, something that would comfort him. "I used to think a good day was when everything went exactly my way," I told him. "I still believe that to be completely happy it takes willingness to learn from the mistakes you make along the way. I've learned that the process of mistake-making might be life-changing: It could be good, it might be bad. It's usually hard to know how things are going to turn out when you start any journey."

He didn't say anything. It was as if Ben hadn't heard me at all. Instead of responding to me, he reached over and grabbed the steering wheel, shaking it violently. His eyes were wide and he looked scary. "There's an army coming out of the radio," he suddenly announced. "I'm starting to feel funny," he said, even louder.

"OK, OK," I said. "Calm down. "I'm not leaving you."

He started to sob and I leaned over to hug him. I don't know how long we sat in the car like that. We just sat until it felt all right to get out, and then we went into the hospital together. After more evaluations and one more CAT scan, the doctors determined nothing had changed inside his head, but they wanted to try out a new medication. He was going to be the guinea pig.

The doctors were reassuring; they told me not to worry. Ben would get used to it in time, they said. He spent one night in the hospital and then slept for several days. He seemed reserved and quiet. He lost his job at the restaurant as a result of not telling them where he was for five days. Then one morning he was up early. Already dressed, he woke me up. "I need to go downtown this morning," he said.

I opened my eyes and looked at the clock on my bedside stand. It said 7:37a.m.. I rolled over on my side, away from him. "When do you need to leave?" I asked.

"Ten minutes," he said.

I got up slowly, pulled a pair of pants and a clean shirt out of my closet, and was ready in no time at all. "I'll buy you coffee, Mom," Ben offered as I drove him to the interview at the new restaurant. He was supposed to talk with the owner about working in the kitchen there. I had to give him credit for his ability to bounce back. It hadn't been even two weeks since our trip to the hospital.

While I waited for him, I made calculations on a pad of paper I always carried with me. One thing was crystal-clear to me that morning: Ben needed his own car. I couldn't keep being his chauffeur. I wanted my life back. Several days earlier, I had been complaining about having to drive Ben all over the place, and a co-worker gave me the name of someone who sold cars cheap. "You need to have car insurance and five hundred dollars cash up front to get a car," she said. "No credit checks either." After that it was one hundred dollars a month.

It sounded almost too good to be true. The problem was, Ben had lousy credit and mine was used up. That made it hard to purchase a car without a huge down payment. The monthly payments were always more than he (we) could afford. I had written the phone number on a scrap of paper. I pulled it from my jacket pocket and dialed the number on my cell phone. A man answered.

"Jimbo's cars," he said. "What can I do for ya?"

"Do you really sell cars for five hundred dollars down?" I asked.

"I do," he replied. "But you can put more down if you'd like. Takes less time to pay back the loan that way."

"And you don't need to have good credit?" I asked.

"What's that?" he said and laughed.

"What happens if someone doesn't make their payments?" I asked.

"Miss," he said. "In all the 25 years I've been in this business I've only had two people skip out on me. I ain't worried about it, my brother-in-law's a cop," he added.

"You're kidding?"

"Miss, are you calling about buying a car or just to talk? Cause I ain't got all day," he said.

"I'm sorry," I said. "What are your hours?"

"Mornings from ten to one, and if you drive over here right now you're gonna see ol' Jimbo's got a car for just about anybody's pocket book," he said, and hung up.

I thought this over for about 30 seconds before reaching into my purse. I pulled out my wallet so I could look at the bank book again. There was over eight hundred dollars in my account. I had saved money all summer long and now I could do it. I could spare five hundred dollars. I had noticed a bank machine on the wall of the shopping center. I looked down at my watch. Ben had been inside the restaurant for nearly 15 minutes; I figured he might be a little longer, so I walked across the parking lot to the ATM and inserted my card. After extracting the five hundred in cash, I went back to the car to wait for Ben.

Pretty soon he came out of the restaurant, and he was smiling. He waved as he made his way across the parking lot, and then gave me a thumbs-up. Ben opened the door and jumped into the passenger seat.

"I got the job!" he said. "And I can start this afternoon."

"We're going to get you a car first," I replied.

"Right now?" he asked, looking puzzled.

I pulled the cash out of my wallet and waved it at him. It was all in twenties, and it spread out like an oriental fan.

"You're crazy," he said.

"I know," I said. "But I'm in charge."

The weeks flew by. Once Ben got his car, I was more or less

freed from my maternal responsibilities again. I had thought about taking a much-needed vacation once August arrived, and then I changed my mind. I had started working with a new group at the geriatrics hospital, all people from the psych unit. They were there for acute care.

It was a strange place indeed.

To begin with, it was a lock-down unit; nobody could enter without knowing the door code, and the patients couldn't leave, although a lot of them tried. Right inside the unit was a long counter, a nurses' station that separated the patients from the outside world. It was staffed by numerous doctors, nurses, and a couple of social workers, all of whom seemed to be very busy filing out paperwork.

Just past the nurses' station was a fairly wide common area with a table in the middle, surrounded by ten rooms that radiated off the main one like spokes of a wheel. There were usually two patients to a room, most of them rotating out every couple of weeks. This wasn't the ideal setting to begin any kind of therapy, much less art therapy, because nobody was around long enough to finish anything that took longer than an hour.

Aside from a daily exercise program the therapeutic recreation department provided, my art therapy session was the only other activity they participated in all week long. As you can well imagine, these people were not just mentally and emotionally challenged, they were depressed and lethargic as well. Their main therapy program appeared to be strictly pharmaceutical in nature. As a result, many of my patients were drowsy or shook uncontrollably from anti-psychotic medications. Some were held down by restraints that kept them from getting up or falling down.

I came on a weekly basis because I was initially interested in finding out more about mental disorders. This seemed like a good place to do that. It was also vaguely similar to the mental hospital where Ben had stayed. I remembered the Christmas tree he had helped to decorate only a few months earlier. Here the options weren't a whole lot better than his had been; patients were either transferred out to long-term care facilities as dementia patients or they were sent home. I never did get the courage to ask the social workers what happened if there wasn't a home to go back to. I didn't think I could stand it if I knew the rest of the story. I just kept coming back to be with them.

Once I got there I would get out all the paint and start to put blank pieces of paper down on the table. Usually they painted pictures — simple landscapes and bowls of flowers mostly. The activity guy, Tommy, always helped me. Nearly every week he would say that nobody was in the mood to do anything that day. Today wasn't any different. Tommy met me inside the door, and I followed him over to the table where I usually set up. "They all seem to be pretty sleepy today," he said. "They're all in their rooms."

One lady sitting at the table was still eating her lunch, even though it was two in the afternoon. The tables were sticky, and there were several ratty-looking magazines on them. I moved these to one side and looked around to find a clean space to put down the paint, but there wasn't any place that was clean. A couple of nursing assistants were standing around watching, but neither of them budged from where they stood to help us. I looked over at Tommy, then back to the nursing assistants.

"They're on break," he said, reading my thoughts.

"Great," I said. "You'll have to clean the tables then."

In the meantime several of the patients had noticed my arrival. The ones who weren't tied down had started to amble toward the table where I was putting out the paint. The woman who was still eating stayed put and looked up at me.

"Get me another cup of tea," she demanded.

I stopped what I was doing long enough to answer her. "Sorry," I said. "I'm not your aide."

"What are you then?" she asked.

"I'm the art therapist," I said. "Would you like to paint?" She shook her head.

"I ain't done with my lunch yet," she said.

Meanwhile Tommy had gotten back with some damp paper

towels; he started using these to clean off the tables. As he wiped them down, we talked. "You're kind of like the circus coming to town up here," he said. "Everybody notices when you're here." His comment caused me to smile.

"What else do they do here all day?" I asked. He shrugged.
"I evaluate them," he said.
"You evaluate them for what?" I asked.
"Oh you know," he told me. "To see if their meds are working or not." I swore under my breath, thinking how would he know?

"What did you say?" he asked. I ignored this question and continued to get out the paint and a coffee can filled with paint brushes. "Just round them up, Tommy," I said.

Pretty soon Tommy had seven or eight people seated around the table. I say seven or eight because they were always getting up and down. Some stayed for the entire time and others came and went. Somebody always had a peculiar request. That day one resident named Susan told me she couldn't sit too close to the table. "I'm claustrophobic," she explained.

I looked around the room. "It's a pretty big room," I said, pushing her a little closer to the table, but she was strong. Susan shoved the chair she was sitting in about two feet backward with one good push. "I told you, I'm not painting," she explained, then she said, "And, I've got to go to the bathroom."

"You're excused," I said.

Meanwhile I surveyed the room. I was looking for Jack. He had been in the psych unit much longer than most; about four weeks. "Where's Jack?" I asked Tommy. He pointed to my right. "In his room, I guess," he told me.

I decided to see for myself. Everybody seemed to be getting along just fine, so I took a moment and walked over to Jack's room. I poked my head in the door. He was sitting on his bed, head in his hands. Poor Jack was shaking and crying. I cleared my throat and waited. He looked up.

"Hi Jack," I said. "Do you want to come out and paint with me?" First he looked confused and didn't answer. Then he shook his head back and forth before he dropped it back into his hands again. I stood there for a moment, but he didn't look up again. It was heartbreaking to see him like that. I said a silent prayer, *Please God, take care of him.* I really didn't know who else would.

I went back to where the others were painting and stood next to Tommy. "What's going on with him?" I asked. I gestured toward Jack's room. Tommy raised his eyebrows, and then went on to explain. "We haven't gotten his meds straightened out yet," he said.

"But he's upset. He's all by himself and he's crying," I said. This time it was Tommy's turn to sigh. He looked away for a minute and then back at me. "Look," he said. "I don't make up the rules, I just work here. We aren't supposed to get involved with them."

"Why is he shaking that much?" I asked. "Does he have Parkinson's?"

"It's the anti-psychotic medication," Tommy said.

At this remark I only nodded because I was thinking of my Ben. I was remembering the doctor telling me he would get used to his medication in time, then Ben crying and telling me he couldn't do it. But he did do it. We had done it together, that's how. And then I remembered why I had come here.

They needed me.

Chapter 13

October 15, 2000

Linda Sue, Richard, Jen, Jen's mom, Carolyn, and I had all gone out to the country together for my plein-air class. We came to a pasture overlooking the valley. It was beautiful and warm outside. High overhead cumulous clouds were floating by, and in the next field a farmer had begun to harvest his corn crop. We set up our easels underneath an old maple tree that grew alongside a small stream. Some of the leaves in the surrounding countryside had started to change, and this tree's leaves were rust colored. We could see other trees in the same field that had turned yellow and orange.

Linda Sue, Jen, and I decided to paint under the maple tree mainly because we preferred shade. Even though it was October, the weather was still quite warm. While the three of us were setting up, Richard tramped off downstream. He was wearing a cowboy hat and an old flannel shirt, and the effect was charming. I was a little sorry to see him go. Jen's mom unfolded a chair she had brought along, set it near us, and got out a book. She settled herself happily and turned a page.

"What are you doing?" I asked. She looked up and smiled serenely.

"I just prefer to read today," she said.

"But you've paid me to teach you how to paint," I pointed out. "And you've come all the way out here. Why are you reading?" She put the book down in her lap, opened to keep her place, and looked thoughtful for a moment or two.

"Then I am paying for the privilege of your company today," Carolyn said, and went back to her book. I shrugged.

"Suit yourself," I said. She looked up again.

"Thank you."

I turned around to see what Jen and Linda Sue were doing. Linda Sue's painting had blown off her easel and landed face-down in the grass. She was bending over, attempting to dislodge it from where it had fallen. She looked up as I made my way to help her.

"Why do things always fall face-down?" she asked.

"Your canvas is heavier on one side because of the paint on it," I told her. "The same thing would have happened if you'd dropped a slice of bread with peanut butter on it."

She held the canvas up for me to see.

"It's ruined," she complained. I agreed with her about that. Grass was stuck to the front of the canvas, and when she tried to pick it off, little indentations were left behind in the paint. "You can always start again," I suggested. Instead Linda Sue threw the painting down.

"I hate it now," she said. "I think I'll go see what Richard's doing." She laid the painting by the trunk of the maple tree.

"It might fall down again," I suggested.

"Who cares?" she said. She tossed her head and turned; she began making her way across the field.

"Where are you going?" I yelled.

"I already told you, to visit Richard," she yelled back. "He looks lonely down there all by himself."

I watched her walk across the field toward him. She looked gorgeous. Linda Sue was wearing an extremely short pair of cut-off jeans and a little white t-shirt. A small section of her stomach showed; it was flat. Her long brown hair blew with the wind as she walked; it seemed to wave goodbye to me. I continued to watch her, so I saw Richard when he looked up. He was smiling broadly as she came closer. I watched them embrace and hug from the distance.

I turned away. Jen was standing in front of an easel, hand on hip, head cocked to one side. On her right I could make out a large area of the canvas. What was there looked a lot like the hedgerow at the far end of the field. Otherwise it wasn't a landscape yet. She must have heard me approaching because suddenly she turned around. From the look on her face, I could see she wasn't pleased with what she had painted.

"It's terrible," she moaned.

I secretly agreed with her. The newly sketched painting, like its creator, lacked perspective. I looked at it again, wondering what I could say to help her improve it. Jen wasn't a natural artist, she was someone who needed an outlet. I knew her mother was dying again — not from the cancer, but from an innate inability to enjoy her own life. She seemed to live vicariously through her daughter or the books she read constantly. What do you say to someone who is suffering?

"It's not that bad," I said. "I think it's a good start," I lied to her.

Jen took a tentative step toward me. "Do you really think so?" she asked. I nodded vigorously and looked at the painting again. What it might have lacked in perspective it certainly made up for in style. Even I had to admit that the hedgerow was especially well drawn in. I pointed this out, mostly because it was the only thing I could think of to say.

"You're a genius," I said. "I love how you sketched the hedgerow in with a strong horizontal line. Once you start to add color, it will help to define the background area. It's a great start," I added for effect. Then I stopped talking and waited to see how she would react to my critique. To my great relief she was smiling.

"Do you mind if I show you something?" I asked. I grabbed her palette and looked up at the sky to study the cumulous clouds. Taking a dab of the ultramarine blue on her palette, I mixed it with zinc white and a little linseed oil. I applied this blue tone to the sky area before going over it again with more zinc white. Continuing in this manner, I was able to form a billowy cloud. Jen looked up at the sky with renewed interest.

"Notice the cloud's darker underside," I pointed out, adding more blue to the bottom of the cloud formation I'd just created. I handed the brush back to her. Jen took it in her left hand and waved it over her head like a baton. During this happy display, Carolyn looked up from her book and clapped her hands with delight.

"Nice, nice, very nice," she exclaimed.

Relieved that I had at least steered Jen away from a painting crisis, I congratulated myself before turning around to see Richard and Linda Sue coming back across the field together. They were laughing and talking. They looked as if they had been best friends forever. I stood where I was and watched them as they approached.

"You forgot to bring your painting," I said.

"Just came back to get a soda out of the car," Richard said. He continued walking toward the road where we had parked his Suburban truck. He climbed the split-rail fence, jumped down, and sauntered over toward the car. Linda Sue stayed behind and motioned excitedly.

"He asked me out," she whispered.

"You're kidding," I said.

"No, I'm not kidding. He asked me out to dinner."

"Where are you going?"

"To that new French restaurant in the city," she said.

I know it was being silly, but I was suddenly envious of her and angry with him. I didn't say anything at first. I just stood there dumbfounded, thinking that he was *my* friend. He had no business asking her out! She had plenty of other male friends, and she could go out with one of them.

"It's not right," I said.

"What do you mean?" she asked, looking puzzled

"I don't date your friends," I said.

"I wouldn't care if you did," she replied. "I don't understand why you're so upset all of a sudden. He's asked you out before, and you turned him down several times."

"Shut up," I said. "He's coming back."

Richard was indeed striding back across the field toward us. In both hands he carried a small cooler, whistling and smiling as he approached. He dropped the cooler on the ground.

"Soda anyone?" he asked nonchalantly.

I folded my arms across my stomach and took a step backward. "Not for me," I said. "But she could probably use some cooling down." I pointed at Linda Sue. He looked up and frowned slightly before pulling out a can of soda. Richard looked at Linda Sue and then back to me.

"Everything OK here?" he asked.

"Everything is perfect," I said.

"Good," he said. "Then I'm going to keep on painting. See you two later." He strode off, leaving the cooler of soda on the ground between Linda Sue and me. We resumed our conversation.

"What's your problem?" she hissed.

"He's still married," I told her.

"He's been separated for nearly three months now; he's not a monk for crying out loud, and he's divorcing his wife."

"Then have a nice time," I said abruptly. "Now can we get back to work?" Linda Sue went back to where she had left her painting and picked it up.

"You're jealous," she replied.

We spent the rest of the afternoon in silence. The class had been together long enough for everyone to feel comfortable painting on their own without a running commentary from me. I was thankful that I could be outside without a lot of interruptions, although Jen's mom took her glasses off at one point and looked directly at me. She had a certain psychic ability that sometimes gave me the creeps.

"You're the one he really likes," Carolyn said, and went back to her reading.

The class painted for another couple of hours while the farmer went on with his harvest. Several Holstein cows approached us tentatively from behind a barbed-wire fence that separated the pasture where we painted from the one where they grazed. It was a lovely country day that only a complete fool wouldn't have appreciated, but I remained glum and morose for the better part of the afternoon. When I finally looked down at my watch, it was four o'clock.

"Let's wrap it up," I yelled out at nobody in particular.

They all came running with everyone gathered almost immediately. Richard was the first one to show me his painting. Linda Sue, Jen, and Carolyn stood off to one side. I held his painting up for them to see.

"It's pretty," Jen said.

After critiquing everybody's work, I made a surprise announcement that the class was now officially over. It was the end. I knew this was abrupt. I knew that they might think something was wrong. I went on to explain that fall had arrived and before long it would be too cold to paint outside. That wasn't the real reason. I had had a sort of epiphany that afternoon. I realized I was sick and tired of being in charge, trying to sound like I knew everything about art or anything else. I felt defeated and incomplete for some reason I couldn't quite identify right then. What I wanted to do was go home and put my head under the covers — or in the oven.

The problem was I didn't know where my home was anymore. Somewhere between college and the present, the idea of home had gotten lost in my life. Things had not worked out in the country with Evelyn. I didn't think of the tiny apartment I now shared with Ben in the suburbs as home, either. I had moved so many times during the past year that I didn't even know where all the grocery stores were yet, let alone feel as if I were part of a community. As Richard drove us all back into town, I stared out the window at the rolling Maryland countryside and wondered where I was going.

He dropped us off at the Starbucks café where we had met

earlier. I let the others unload their easels and canvases before getting my stuff out of his car. While I waited for them to unload, he put his hand on my shoulder. We stood together like that for a minute or two. His hand felt warm on my shoulder, but his presence only made me feel worse. In my mind I was still an orphan.

"What's wrong?" he asked. I shrugged his hand off.

"Nothing," I said, pulling back. And then I said, "I don't want you to call me anymore." He looked shocked. He even looked like he might cry. But that wasn't possible. He had just asked my friend out to dinner.

"I thought *we* were friends," he said.

"We are, but I don't appreciate you using my art class as a dating service," I said. A glimmer of understanding quickly crossed his face.

"Oh," he said. "I hope you know I'm not that attracted to her."

"If you're interested in dating lots of people," I retorted, "just leave me out of it."

I pulled my knapsack out of his car and threw my easel over my shoulder before turning around. I left him standing there. I walked back across the parking lot to my car, opened the trunk with a violent jerk, and threw my stuff in. Richard followed right along behind me, but I pretended to ignore him.

"Do you want to get a cup of coffee?" he asked. He gestured towards Starbucks. I shook my head and let the trunk slam shut.

"No," I said. He started to smile at me, and then stopped himself.

"How come?" he asked.

"Because I hate you, that's why," I said, opening my car door. I got behind the wheel and started the ignition.

He stepped back from the car. I guess I must have scared him throwing my gear around and slamming the trunk shut. I drove out of the parking lot, but I had to stop before pulling onto the street. At that moment I looked look back at him in the rearview mirror. He looked sad. I thought about him all the way home and every day after that.

October 17, 2000

Gertrude was sitting at her card table when I arrived. I was running late because Irene had stopped me on my way up the stairs to deliver a graphic description of how she had cleaned up after the dog that morning. She stood in the hallway, leaning over the banister.

"That dog has shit on the floor again." Irene said.

"I'm sorry," I told her, trying to look sympathetic.

Irene pointed down the hall toward Gertrude's room. The dishrag in her hand drooped like a flag without any wind. "It's because of that useless invalid in there. She feeds that stupid thing off her plate, and they let her get away with it, too."

"I can't imagine," I said.

She raised her eyebrows to convey that I hadn't comprehended the magnitude of her statements. "It's downright *disgusting* if you ask me," she said.

"Where is the dog now?" I asked.

Irene looked surprised. She put her hand over her mouth and spoke through her fingers. "Oh, my God, I forgot to bring him inside!" She pushed me out of the way and lumbered down the stairs. "Damn thing, it's all her fault, too," she said. I waited until I heard the front door slam before I knocked and entered Gertrude's room.

"I'm having a bad day," Gertrude said after I had shut the door.

She didn't turn around but continued speaking to me. "Make sure you lock the door so that nasty woman won't come in here again," she said. "She's been on the rampage all morning."

"I know," I said. "I just ran into her in the hall."

Gertrude patted the metal chair beside her. It was her signal for me to sit down. I got the painting we had been working on the week before and examined it. "This is coming along nicely," I told her. Then I sat down at the table and positioned the painting in front of her, looking around for the paint box.

"Where'd the paint get off to?" I asked.

"She probably stole it," Gertrude answered. She leaned closer and dropped her voice to a whisper. "You know *who*, right?"

"Don't worry," I said. "She's got a project going right now. I doubt she'll be bothering us."

I stood up then and opened the top drawer of the dresser she referred to as her cupboard.

Sure enough, tucked in with the stockings and handkerchiefs was the paint box. Underneath the paint box there was a small pile of crackers wrapped in plastic foil. I pulled everything out and set it all on the card table in front of Gertrude.

"The Mrs. doesn't like it when you stash food in the drawers," I said. Gertrude reached over and patted my hand, as if to reassure me.

"It's all right," she said. "I save the crackers for Scout. He comes up every day and helps me eat my lunch."

Inwardly I laughed, thinking of Irene having to clean up after Scout, but I kept that image to myself. Instead I opened up the paint box and got up to go into the bathroom for a glass of water. When I came back, Gertrude was already scratching her head, holding her painting up in the light.

"I'm going to give this one to my daughter," she said. "It reminds me of the time when my husband Frank went to war. Jane was only a little girl then. I'd take her out to the backyard where he set up a swing in the tree before he left to go overseas. My Frank told me to take our girl out every day and get her some exercise."

The painting we had been working on depicted a woman in a broad-brimmed hat sitting in a chair and holding a baby. There was a tree in the background and a picket fence beyond the tree. "There's no swing in the tree, Gertrude," I said.

"Doesn't need to be," she said. She sat back in her wheelchair and gazed dreamily out the window. "Every time I took her out to play she would swing in that tree. She liked to swing, and I'd think about my Frank." Gertrude stopped and took a hanky from her sleeve. She wiped her eyes and went on talking. "He was the kindest man that ever lived," she said.

"Was it hard?" I asked.

"Everything was hard during the war," she said. "We didn't have a car, and I lived in two rooms in Mrs. McCready's house while he was gone. I shared the upstairs bathroom with Mrs. McCready."

"I mean did you miss him?"

"That goes without saying," she said. "He was gone four long years, and I missed him every day just as much as the first day he left."

"How did you know he was the one?" I asked.

Gertrude looked confused. "What do you mean by that?" she said.

I cleared my throat. "I mean, after you met Frank, how did you know you loved him?"

"Well, I didn't know at first," she explained. "I was going with another guy named Billy Smith when I first met him. Frank was playing baseball for the public school, and I tagged along with my sister to the game. Her beau was playing for St. Joseph's High, and she didn't want to go by herself. When I first saw him, he was standing on first base getting ready to run, and I asked my sister who that guy was, but she didn't know."

"How did you finally meet him?" I said.

Gertrude scratched her head. "That came later," she replied. "But I went home after the game and asked my grandfather."

"Asked him what?"

"I asked him if it was all right to break up with a guy you'd been seeing for a while to take a chance on somebody else," she said.

"What did he say?"

"He wanted to know if Frank was a Catholic," she said.

"Was he?"

"Mercy no, he was a Baptist," she said, laughing.

I began adding water to her paint cubes in the box. I got a

dab of hunter's green paint on the brush and handed it to Gertrude. "Let's see if you can take this color and fill in the lawn area," I said. I leaned over and outlined where the lawn would be, then I sat back in my chair to watch her paint. Gertrude began to paint in the lawn; we didn't speak for another minute or so. After she had finished the lawn, she sat back in her wheelchair and picked up the conversation where we had left off.

"I just kept going back to watch him play ball," she said. "Before long he asked me for a date."

"Then what happened?" I asked.

"Well, we kept on seeing one another after the games for ice cream sodas, and one time I went with him to see a movie. But I was still officially going out with Billy so I talked to my grandfather about it."

"What did you want to know?" I asked.

"If it was OK to break up with one to go out with the other," she said.

"And what did he say?"

"I'll never forget that day," she said. "My grandfather was sitting in his favorite chair in the parlor. He had just filled his pipe and was lighting it as I came into the room. He looked up and saw me and said 'Something's on your mind, girl,' and then he motioned for me to sit down. So I settled down on the braided rug in front of his chair, and he took a puff on his pipe."

"'What's the matter with my girl?' Grandfather asked me. He blew a smoke ring, and I watched it expand and fill up the room," Gertrude said. I moved around in my chair. I wanted to hear what advice her grandfather had given Gertrude that day.

"I asked him if it was a sin to want to go out with Frank after I'd been engaged to Billy," she said. "But instead of responding, he asked me a question," Gertrude said. I leaned closer now so I could hear exactly what he had asked her. The painting was quite forgotten.

"He asked me, 'Do you love Frank?' I said yes. And he said, 'Then that's your answer.' So it was simple after that. I told Billy I couldn't see him anymore and gave him his ring back."

"How did you know you loved Frank?" I said.

Gertrude smiled at me. "Because every time I was with Billy, I was thinking about Frank," she said.

Chapter 14

April 24, 2004

I followed the directions the Professor had given me to the convalescent center where Gertrude was staying. It was mid-afternoon, and the parking lot was full. It had rained earlier, but the sun had just started to come out again. I drove around for several minutes, hoping that someone would pull out, but in the end I parked illegally in the staff lot behind one of the main buildings. I knew from experience that no one would notice or care.

The facility was being expanded and renovated. Tall mounds of dirt and jumbles of wire fencing lay around the borders of the buildings. I could hear the drone of large engines somewhere in the background. Everything was busy, busy, busy. People were coming and going into the building from the street level, and I followed a small group into the lobby area. Inside, a large sign indicated where everything was located. It was all very confusing. I looked at this information for a few moments and then went to the reception desk. A very bored-looking woman glanced up from a book and absently asked me, "What you need?"

"I need to locate the long-term care unit," I said. "I'm here to see a patient."

"Where she at?" the receptionist asked.

"I just told you, the special care unit."

She pointed over her shoulder without even looking at me and said, "Over there, take that elevator to the second floor."

I managed to get on the next elevator going up and got off on the second floor. I ended up asking for more directions from two other people before I finally found Gertrude's room. I maneuvered down several hallways and around one nurse's station before I found her. The entire area was dark and gloomy despite the restoration that was going on. I wondered if they were going to turn on the lights. Was it always this dark in here? It reminded me of the first time I had met Gertrude, when I had walked down the hallway to her room at the Professor's house. How dismal her hallway had been there, too. It seemed it had all happened a very long time ago; the thought saddened me now. The door to her room was ajar, and I could see Gertrude sitting up in a chair.

She was dressed, and her hair had been combed flat against her head. She looked different than I remembered. For one thing, she was wearing clothes, and the nightcap was missing. In all the years we had been together, I had seen her only in a nightdress or bathrobe.

She was staring straight ahead and didn't turn when I entered her room. The overhead light was off, but there was a large window on one side of the room, and the shade had been raised. I could see and hear a tree's branches scraping against the pane of glass; there were large pink buds at the end of each branch. Otherwise the little room was devoid of ornament. There was a small cot, a nightstand, and, of course, the chair that Gertrude was sitting in.

I stepped gingerly in front of Gertrude, but she didn't seem to realize I was there. She continued to stare straight ahead. Her eyes were glazed over, and she held a small towel that she kept putting up to her mouth. My eyes had adjusted to the light now and I saw why she was using the towel. Gertrude was drooling.

"Hi, Gertrude, it's me."

I startled her at first, but she began to squint and look me up and down, keeping the towel near her mouth the whole time. She didn't say anything, so I tried again.

"Do you remember me?" I asked. She nodded her head yes.

"Paint." she said.

"Yes, we paint together. I'm your art teacher," I explained.

She smiled, and I saw that her dentures had been removed. She was smiling up with pink gums and catching little rivulets of drool with the towel. The sight of her like this actually sickened me for a moment. She must have sensed my chagrin, because suddenly tears came into her eyes, and she made an effort to speak again. She took the towel away from her face.

"I'm sorry," she said.

"Oh, God, don't," I said. Then I dropped down on my knees in front of her, putting my hands into her lap. We were both crying now.

Finally I gathered myself and straightened up a bit. She was still holding my hands in hers, searching my face. My knees were going numb, but I stayed where I was. The linoleum where I had been kneeling was shiny and very hard. I looked around the room again. I noticed that the bare walls had been painted a neutral tan. I wiped my eyes with the side of one hand that I had extracted from Gertrude's clutch. "We'll have to hang some of your paintings up," I said.

She nodded in agreement as she looked around her room.

"Where am I?" she asked.

"You're at a long-term care facility," I explained. You'll be staying here until you can go home again." I knew that this was a boldfaced lie, but I couldn't bear to tell her that she would probably die here. Gertrude shook her head back and forth.

"No," she said.

"Yes, you will, Gertrude, you'll go home again soon."

"Troy Hill?" she asked.

I knew that she was referring to her lifelong home near Pittsburgh. Gertrude had told me numerous stories over the years about what her life had been like there, living in a row house three doors down the street from St. Anthony's Cathedral. The church was famous for its stations of the cross — scenes with life-sized statues depicting the passion of Jesus.

Busloads of people came from all over the United States to see the Stations of the Cross there. Many of the visitors had touched the statue of Jesus over the years, wearing some of the patina off his features. Eventually an alarm system had been installed to prevent this from happening, but every so often Gertrude would hear the alarm going off, and then she would exclaim, "Somebody's touching Jesus again!" She loved to tell me that particular story, over and over again.

During our time together, she had told me many stories about her life and her family. Her real father had died of influenza in 1918, leaving her mother to take care of four small children. They had moved in with Gertrude's grandfather, and her mother had taken a job as a cook with a wealthy family in town. Within two years her mother had remarried a man who had lost his wife in the same influenza epidemic. He had been left with two young children, now combined with the four from Gertrude's family. Eventually they had two more children together, which made a grand total of eight mouths to feed, eight bodies to clothe.

I used to question how they had managed, but Gertrude always described her life as happy, filled with escapades with her brothers and sisters. She never once spoke of herself as impoverished; instead, she had been rich with family, church, and God in her life. When we painted, she would always say to me, "Make it good!" That phrase was one that her grandfather had instilled in her from the time she was a little girl. She told me that was her motto in life, and she felt obliged to pass it on to me.

"If you do your best, you'll come out all right, no matter what," she would tell me. And then she would point her index finger straight up, adding "and don't forget to pray."

I wondered how she would describe her life now. I also wondered if anyone would answer her last question truthfully. It was obvious that she was never going home again, not to her son's home and definitely not to Troy Hill. I looked around her room again, at the empty walls and the hard linoleum floor. The tree outside was scratching at the window, bringing me back to the present. I had lied to her.

All these years, my job has been to convince people who are suddenly hospitalized, dying, or disabled that they have something to live for, and for the last ten years or so I have done just that. I have transformed invalids and people with Alzheimer's disease into artists; the lame paint, the blind sing, and they do so right up until the day they die. Now I didn't know what I was going to say or do. Suddenly I had an idea. I was going to take Gertrude's advice.

I said a silent prayer. *"Help me, God, to know what to say to her."* As if in answer, God must have spoken through Gertrude right then and there. To my great surprise, she asked another question.

"How is your life?"

The funny thing was that in all the years we had known each other, she had never once asked me about my life. She had always seemed more interested in telling her own stories, and I had let her. The other truth was, she simply knew very little, if anything about me at all.

"My son Ben graduates from college this spring," I said. At this she nodded, as if to tell me she approved.

"Did you get married?" she asked.

"Yes, about two years ago."

Gertrude smiled. She waved her hand toward the door. "Then you can go home now," she said.

She closed her eyes and lay back in her chair. I waited a minute or two, but she looked as if she had gone to sleep. I stood up gradually and turned to look down at her for the last time. She looked peaceful, just like a saint should.

The End